The Big Book of Herbal Medicine

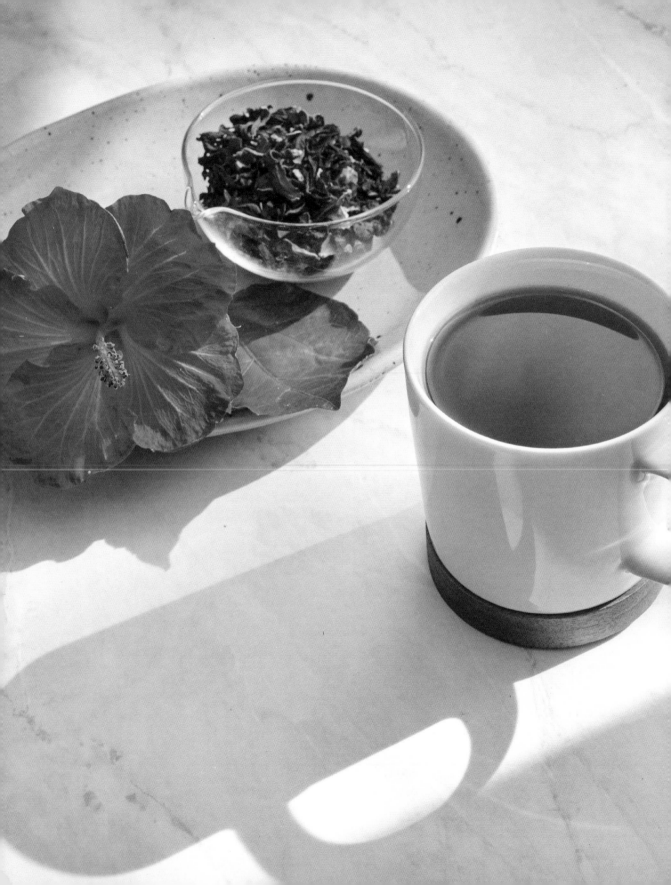

The *The* **BIG** **BOOK** *of* **HERBAL** **MEDICINE**

300 Natural Remedies for Health and Wellness

TINA SAMS

Photography by Marija Vidal

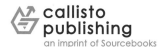

callisto publishing
an imprint of Sourcebooks

Published by Callisto Publishing LLC C/O Sourcebooks LLC
P.O. Box 4410, Naperville, Illinois 60567-4410
(630) 961-3900
callistopublishing.com

Printed and bound in China
OGP 2

With deep gratitude to all the elders who have gone before us, keeping the knowledge alive.

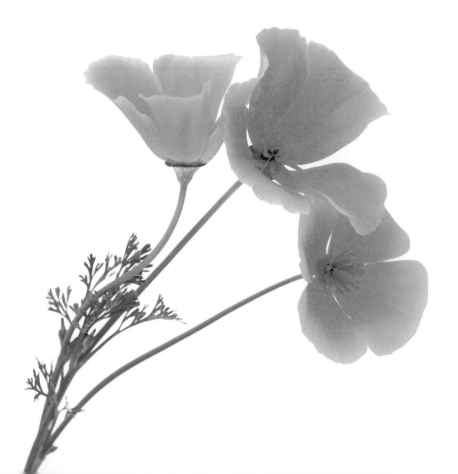

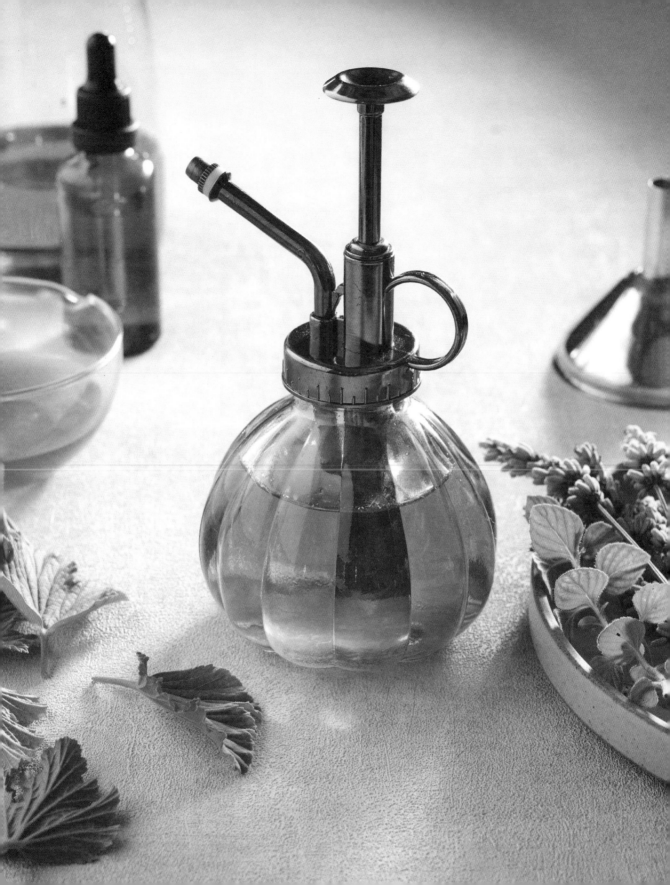

CONTENTS

Introduction

I am bursting with excitement to share this book. Herbs have been an immense part of my life (and living) for more than 30 years. There is always some new way to incorporate the enjoyment of herbs into life. For instance, right now, I'm taken with eco-printing plants on fabric, which adds another layer to all the other ways herbs have wound their way around my heart.

As a child, I wandered country roads, learning about butter-and-eggs (*Linaria vulgaris*), chicory, sassafras, alfalfa, plantain, and all the wild roadside plants. They were just part of every day. Eventually, my sister and I were invited to open an herb shop at the local Renaissance festival, and the rest is history. Currently, I edit and publish an herb magazine, talking every single day with other herbalists and herb enthusiasts, keeping my ear to the ground, and paying attention to what people want to know about plants.

No matter what your level of expertise, from beginner to practitioner, there is something here for you. Working with herbs is a humble but important strand in the web of life. We are all connected. Humans, animals, insects, and plants all share this earth, and we're all important to one another. We become more and more aware of this connection as we partake of the herbal medicines we are about to create.

There is such a spectrum of herbal medicine. For some people, it is easier to begin by swapping in herbs for allopathic, or conventional, medicine. That approach is often looked down upon, though nearly everyone starts that way. Eventually, we learn to start listening to our intuition and may choose herbs that way. Many people take note of the plants (usually considered weeds) that are seeking them out and showing up at the door. There are as many ways to approach herbalism as there are people in the world. Do what works for you. Always remember that plant medicine is indeed powerful, and we need to take it seriously. Each of us is different, with our own constitution and health issues, or lack thereof. Herbal medicine should not be added to prescribed pharmaceutical medications without the consultation of medical providers and experienced herbal practitioners.

In the following pages, you will find a solid educational foundation on herbs. You will learn to create all kinds of different herbal healers, like soothing and comforting topical remedies for the skin and joints, aromatics to improve mood or respiration, teas, tinctures, syrups, and salves, and, eventually, you might even decide to try your hand at blending your own concoctions.

In this book, you'll find profiles on 90 different herbs. Most likely, you'll find that a handful of them will suit you 90 percent of the time, but the others may come in handy on rarer occasions. We'll never know all the herbs, but each of us can choose a different handful as our favorites.

There are also 300 remedies and recipes to alleviate or prevent all sorts of ailments.

Soon, you'll be putting on the kettle to make some herbal tea to settle in at night. There will be a jar of cayenne peppers in oil on the shelf, soaking in preparation for the creation of an arthritic knee salve. The bowl on the table will hold bunches of elderberries and echinacea blossoms, soon to be a winter wellness elixir, and that giant bottle of vodka on the counter next to the scavenged jars is waiting to become a series of tinctures from the herbs scheduled to arrive in the mail this afternoon (or gathered from the garden this morning). The bed in the guest room is probably covered by an extra sheet full of drying blossoms. Such is the life of the herbal medicine maker.

Now more than ever, we need to learn about the plants around us and reacquaint ourselves with the knowledge that previous generations gave up in preference to modern medicines. I live in a farming community, and we all have our own niches. My sister lives down the hill, and she's the soap maker. I am the forager and the medicine maker. We have various farmers growing food, a few builders, a mechanic, and so on. The day may come when we need to once again know how to take care of ourselves—and one another—even if it's just during a power outage that lasts a couple of days.

Welcome to the world of herbs! I hope with this book you'll learn another way to make your way in this world.

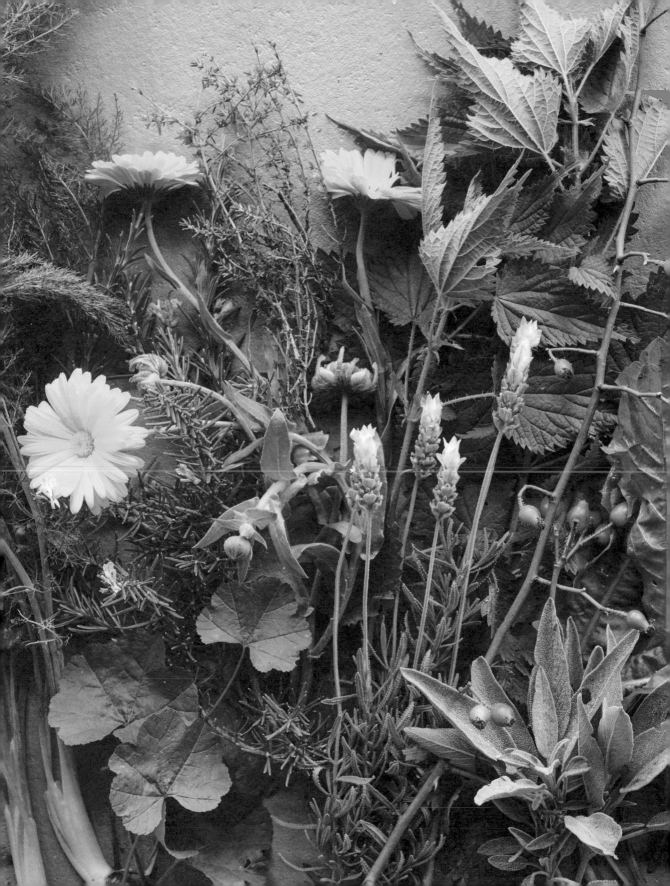

PART ONE

Understanding Herbal Medicine

The use of healing herbs is as old as the hills. All creatures have been observed finding comfort in plants for all kinds of reasons. Domesticated dogs and cats munch on grass to settle their stomachs. We all seek shade under trees, and after a long, hard winter, the first glimpse of green, or (gasp!) a flower, takes our breath away.

Modern society looked away for a while, fixating on new, synthetic, and packaged solutions to our problems, but in the last few decades there has been a renaissance of herbalism as we seek a reconnection to nature to balance our cyber-centered lives. The wonder of it is that Nature has been waiting to share her gifts with us.

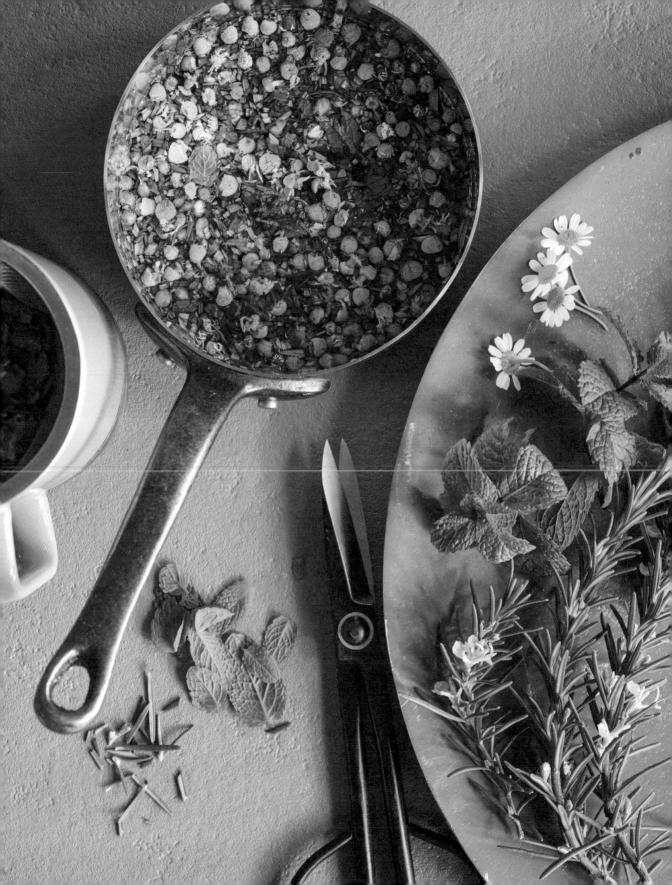

CHAPTER ONE

What Is Herbal Medicine?

There is a rich and fascinating history of herbal medicine and our approach to it. Throughout time, herbs have been considered miracles, witchcraft, and simple ingredients for home remedies. Their legality has been questioned because they have been seen as either dangerous or worthless. Their power is illustrated clearly by this history.

Now, we can easily obtain herbs, whether we grow them, forage them, find them at shops, or order them online. There has never been a better time to learn to work with herbs to help yourself and your loved ones remain happy and healthy.

Healing Herbs

So, you're probably wondering by now: What are the healing herbs and what can they do? The truth is that many of them are probably already stashed in your kitchen somewhere. Take chamomile or mint tea—both are healing herbs! Knowing just three or four herbs and their properties as well as you know that ginger ale helps an upset stomach will make a huge difference in your daily life. There are hundreds of herbal remedies, but here's a taste of a few you might have in (or outside of) your home.

Take oatmeal. It's bulky and keeps us regular, but did you know that it also nourishes the nervous system, helping ease anxiety and stress? Hot peppers, turmeric, and sour cherries are all helpers for the pain of arthritis. Parsley combats bad breath, and those bright green leaves also boost the immune system, stabilize blood sugar, and reduce inflammation. And that oregano on your pizza? It's packed with antioxidants, which help prevent a number of issues related to aging and may even help fight cancer.

It's also important to learn about the weeds outside (and stop killing them with chemicals!) because they can provide surprising benefits. Wild mint (brightens mood), dandelion (protects the liver), yarrow (acts as an antiviral, and relaxes us), St. John's wort (soothes nerves), mimosa (alleviates grief), and goldenrod (fights allergies) are just a few examples of these wonderful healers. Just outside your door, there are likely to be herbs to heal rashes, insect bites, anxiety, excess bleeding, colds and flu, fevers, sore throats, digestive disorders, and so much more. I'll help you navigate these weeds so you can understand their benefits, and I'll give you ideas for other healing plants to cultivate depending on your needs. Let the medicine making begin!

Brief History of Herbal Medicine

2800 BCE: *Shen Nung Pen Ts'ao Ching*, attributed to legendary emperor Shen Nung, is written. This is the first written record detailing the use of herbal medicine.

400 BCE: Greek herbal medicine becomes popular. Hippocrates writes extensively on the topics of diagnosing and treating common illnesses.

50 CE: As the Roman Empire grows, herbal medicine practices spread. Many people begin cultivating herbs for medicinal use.

200: Galen of Pergamon's works are published and popularized. Common illnesses are identified and paired with herbal remedies.

800: Monks become renowned as healers, growing vast herb gardens and transforming many monasteries into infirmaries where sick and injured people are treated in restful surroundings.

900 to 1199: Physician Avicenna pens *The Canon of Medicine*, which mentions many effective herbal remedies. Around the same time, Arab healers gain renown, influencing medical practices.

1347 to 1351: The Black Death sweeps across Europe. Herbal medicines are proven to be as effective as—if not more effective than—common treatments such as bleeding and purging.

1500 to 1599: England's King Henry VII and his Parliament promote trained herbalists, improving the standard of care.

1600 to 1699: Rich patients can afford drugs, which unfortunately come with side effects. The poor are treated with herbal remedies. Around the same time, Nicholas Culpeper's famous herbal book *The English Physician* is published.

1700 to 1799: High-profile Methodist preacher Charles Wesley advocates clean living and promotes herbal treatments for good health.

1800 to 1899: Early pharmaceuticals are developed, but people soon realize that taking drugs leads to side effects, and many return to using herbal remedies. The National Institute of Medical Herbalists is founded in England in 1864.

1900 to 1999: Drug shortages during the First World War lead to a renewed interest in herbal medicine. Interest wanes with the discovery of penicillin. By the 1950s, people look once again to herbal treatments.

2000 to Present: The European Union takes action, regulating and testing herbal medicine in the same fashion as pharmaceuticals. In Europe, herbal medicine enjoys increased popularity and is widely used.

Benefits of Herbal Medicine

Herbs have been a staple of healing in our house for nearly 30 years. When someone has an ailment, I reach for the herbs first—before going to the drugstore, before calling the doctor.

For example, one summer a family member ran over ground bee nests a few different times on his mower (talk about bad luck!). The first two times, he refused to use any herbs and was in pain for days. The third time, he finally let me apply mashed plantain (as a poultice; page 34) to draw out the venom. His pain stopped immediately, and there was no swelling.

During another period in my life, I was caring for a sick sibling who was waiting for an organ transplant. I was warned not to bring any sort of virus or infection into the house because, frankly, it could kill him. For nearly three years, I regularly took elder and holy basil to stay healthy, and they worked. Foods and spices eaten mindfully at the right time can make a huge difference.

The best part? Neither of these treatments cost more than a few dollars. The plantain was growing everywhere—I just had to pick it and mix it with water in the food processor. I grow elder and holy basil in my yard and made them into tinctures (page 32), so vodka was my only expense.

Most herbs are safe and gentle (especially those we use as foods and spices), but remember that they are real medicine and should be treated as such. If you take pharmaceutical medications, talk to your doctor and do your research before using herbs. For instance, lemon balm can negatively affect medications used for thyroid issues. Many herbs also thin the blood, which can cause problems if you're taking a blood thinner. If you develop a rash, swelling, or any new symptom while taking the herb, stop using it immediately.

Aside from being inexpensive, herbal remedies can save you time and money over the long run. With a little forethought and some solid knowledge, herbs make it easy to remain healthy. Simply incorporating them into meals and beverages is a huge step in the right direction. Many herbs have similar functions, so if one isn't convenient or tastes bad, simply exchange it for another.

Most people start by learning how to use herbs to manage symptoms of illnesses that will go away on their own, such as the common cold or respiratory issues. We call those self-limiting illnesses, and they make up a large percentage of (sometimes unnecessary) doctor's visits. We can also learn how to prevent or relieve chronic disease, sometimes even reducing damage already done. I'm not suggesting dismissing traditional medicine altogether; rather, I'm encouraging you to understand your options.

CONVENTIONAL VS. HERBAL MEDICINE

Herbal medicine is different from what many of us are accustomed to with traditional medicine. For instance, when used for chronic or entrenched problems like high blood pressure, gastroesophageal reflux disease (GERD), migraines, or reproductive issues, herbal remedies require time and consistency before you'll notice the effects.

However, for minor issues like colds, cramps, or rashes and skin problems, herbs can be as quickly effective as anything you'll find on the drugstore shelf.

A little-known fact is that lots of drugs are actually derived from herbs. One of the best known is the heart medication digitalis, or digoxin, which comes from the foxglove plant. The cancer drug Taxol comes from Pacific yew trees. Of course, there's codeine from poppies, and aspirin from willows. There's a big difference, though: Pharmaceutical drugs are made by isolating one or two components or chemical constituents from a plant, and then using only those. Pharmaceuticals concentrate that one part of the plant that does that one thing. But plants are so much more than one thing! By contrast, herbal medicine uses all of the components and constituents in the plant, believing that each has a purpose.

It is now quite possible to find a doctor who is learning about herbs and willing to combine them with other medical treatment. I think that's the best of all possible worlds. It is important to get good diagnoses and to see a doctor if a symptom sticks around too long. Don't avoid getting checked out, and always tell your doctor about any herbs you're taking regularly.

How Are Medicinal Herbs Used?

Although medicinal herbs might seem to be the newest thing, in fact they are the oldest thing! As long as time has been recorded, humans have used plants for healing and nutrition.

There is plenty of evidence of herbal healing in the Bible (although the specific plants are often difficult to ascertain). During the Middle Ages, along with bloodletting and leeches, herbs were the only treatments available. During the Civil War, yarrow was a valued styptic (used to stop bleeding), echinacea helped fight infections, pennyroyal was used as an insect repellent, and slippery elm soothed sore throats. As recently as World War II, thyme, foxglove, and peat moss, as well as many other herbs, were purchased from wild crafters who made their living searching woods and meadows for important medicinal plants. There are still people today who harvest wild herbs for a living.

Although other parts of the world found ways to incorporate drugs like penicillin and then the sulfa drugs into their natural healing modalities, Americans dropped herbs like hot potatoes and embraced "better living through chemistry." But in recent decades, people have begun to flock back to herbs in search of the healing knowledge our ancestors took for granted. I remember that my grandfather knew plants only by the nicknames that people from his era used. Even when he didn't know the name, he could go out into the woods or meadows and find a plant that would cure a specific ailment. He had a knack for being able to look at a place and say, "I think the plant will be back in there." I am fortunate to have inherited some of his instincts, which makes it easy to find what I need.

Herbs have thousands of components, more than we will ever identify, and they work together to buffer side effects, potentiate other aspects, and, quite honestly, heal in ways we don't yet understand. Using the whole herbs in preparations, as we'll be learning in the next section, makes them safer and more effective at the same time. All those herbs in your kitchen just waiting to help you will soon become teas, tinctures, elixirs, salves, oils, compresses, and more.

In comparison to pharmaceutical drugs, herbs are extremely safe. The very rare cases of herb-related death are something the entire herb community holds as history. However, mistakes can happen, and deaths have occurred due to overuse and misidentifying herbs that were actually poisonous. Yes, there are poisonous herbs out there, but they are few in number. Herbs labeled as toxic might produce anything from an upset stomach to liver and kidney failure. In more tropical areas, there are more toxic plants. Here are a few things you can do to stay safe:

- Always learn foraging from an expert.

- Research herbs before using them.

- Start at the lowest dose and work up if needed.

WHERE TO GET HERBS

How you obtain your herbs really depends on where you live—the city, the country, or the suburbs—and your lifestyle. But the three ways to collect herbs are to forage, grow your own, or purchase them.

I live in the country, and 80 percent of the herbs I use are wild—also known as weeds! Herbs are plentiful, but being in the country means that there are many conventional farms around me that use chemicals; I pay attention to the farms' locations and when they are spraying, and I stay well away from them. Do not forage herbs that you suspect have been sprayed. In a rural area, hiking trails, unless they are plant conservancies, are safe places to forage and excellent places to learn plant identification.

If you find a safe place to forage, it's important not to gather or taste any herb that you haven't positively identified. Get a couple field guides and study them. Take the field guides and a baggie or basket out into the wild. When an interesting specimen appears, try to determine what the plant is. Take a sprig of it (if there's plenty there) home so you can study it more thoroughly. Once you get a probable ID, put the name of the plant into your browser and do an image search. This will usually tell you if the plant is or isn't what you thought. You don't want to play any guessing games when it comes to foraged plants!

Growing herbs is probably my top choice, and you can do this whether you live on a farm or in a tiny city apartment. You can purchase seeds or starter plants online or at your local nursery. Either way, growing is immensely rewarding.

Another option is purchasing herbs. It's important to use organic herbs in order to avoid chemicals that can be extremely harmful. As consumers, we can use our purchasing power to put an end to the use of these substances that are creating new and ever-more resistant pests and plant diseases, not to mention hurting insects, birds, and animals. Fortunately, there are many organic, sustainable, and environmentally conscious people and companies selling beautiful, high-quality herbs. Good-quality herbs have life in them. They don't look like hay. They have color, scent, and body.

Barks and roots last a couple of years. Aerial herbs—the parts of the herbs that grow aboveground but aren't bark, seeds, or fruit—don't last forever. You can extend their usefulness with proper care, such as keeping them in light-blocking containers and storing them in a cool, dry place. When the herbs no longer look, smell, or feel fresh, it's time for the compost pile. After drying, aerial herbs are considered fresh for about a year if stored well.

Herbal Medicine Today

Today, more than three-quarters of the global population uses herbal medicine. Western researchers have proven in studies what has been passed down through generations for centuries: Plants grown and used at home are effective at treating non-life-threatening diseases and injuries or ailments such as bumps, bruises, headaches, fever, stress, depression, fatigue, and more.

It makes sense. Consider all the plants you eat on a regular basis (yep, the same ones you pull from your garden or the produce section of your favorite grocer): parsley, cilantro, sage, thyme, garlic, basil, ginger, mint. You might toss them in a salad because they add kicks of flavor, but they do double duty once they're inside your body. They carry antioxidants and nutrients that bolster your immune system to fight disease before it starts. In modern doctor's circles, they call that "preventive" medicine. So, why wouldn't those same herbs be used just as successfully for healing after you've gotten sick? St. John's wort looks beautiful in a vase, but it's also fantastic for lowering stress. Chamomile makes a lovely after-dinner tea, or you can use it to relieve indigestion, alleviate muscle spasms, reduce inflammation, or cure infections—talk about getting two (or more) for one!

FAQs about Herbal Medicine

1. Where do medicinal herbs come from?

Some medicinal herbs can be foraged, but most of the botanicals used in herbal medicine are cultivated specifically for health-care purposes. The great news is you can grow your own herbs, but no pressure: If you don't have a green thumb, there are plenty of businesses that sell quality medicinal herbs.

In the United States, herbs are considered dietary supplements. Unlike prescription drugs, they can be sold without first being tested to prove that they are both safe and effective. For this reason, it's smart to be selective about the remedies you try and any herbs you purchase. Unfortunately, there are companies that produce supplements that contain impurities. So, do your homework when you're making decisions about where to buy herbs for medicinal use (or start with the list I've provided in the Resources section of this book, page 382). This will help you not only ensure your safety but also get the best herbs available.

2. Can everyone take herbal remedies?

Some people should use extreme caution when considering herbal remedies. Elderly people tend to metabolize medication differently than younger people do, so if you fall into this category, use herbal treatments cautiously. The same applies to those with immune disorders or anyone who takes prescription drugs. If you are unsure about the safety of an herbal remedy, err on the side of caution and consult a medical professional who is familiar with the proper use of medicinal herbs.

3. Is it safe to make my own herbal remedies?

Nearly everyone can benefit from homemade herbal remedies like those found in this book or other reliable sources (see Resources, page 382). But always make sure to follow any recommended precautions, whether you're compounding a remedy to treat an illness or creating a supplement to increase overall health and well-being.

4. Are herbal medicines sold in stores?

Many high-quality herbal medicines can be found at health-food stores, and there are several reputable online retailers that offer herbal remedies (see Resources, page 382). Tinctures, teas, syrups, liquid extracts, whole herbs, and essential oils are among the most common types of herbal medicines available for sale.

5. Are there any dangers associated with herbal medicines?

Like pharmaceuticals, herbal medicines can be extremely powerful. Although none of the most dangerous herbs are included in this book, some common remedies come with potential hazards. Take the time to learn all you can about the herbs you are interested in using before you start, and take warnings seriously. Some of the most common hazards include drowsiness, sensitivity, allergic reactions, and drug interactions.

6. What types of ailments are herbal medicines used to treat?

The great news about medicinal herbs is that almost every imaginable ailment has an herbal treatment! Even emotional disorders such as anxiety and mild depression can be alleviated with herbal remedies that are used appropriately.

7. Can I grow my own herbal medicines?

Yes! Many herbs can be grown at home. Simply read up on the conditions needed and then determine if you have the right amount of natural sunlight and proper soil conditions available in your garden. You can even grow your own mini herb garden in a sunny spot indoors, so your herbs are right at your fingertips.

8. When should herbal medicines be taken?

Most herbal medicines should be taken at least 30 minutes before or after you eat. If you take vitamins, over-the-counter (OTC) medications, or other herbal remedies, take them two hours apart unless otherwise directed.

9. Is herbal medicine the same as traditional Chinese medicine?

There are some similarities between herbal medicine and traditional Chinese medicine, but they are not the same. In herbal medicine, many treatments consist of the use of single herbs. In traditional Chinese medicine, precise and complex formulas containing up to 15 different herbs are used. Traditional Chinese medicine also includes the use of acupuncture, moxibustion, and other healing techniques.

10. Can children use herbal medicine?

Although children can absolutely enjoy the healing power of herbs, it is important to note that there are herbal remedies that are safe for adults but not safe for children. Herbs and preformulated herbal remedies that are not suitable for children typically come with warnings to that effect. If you ever have a question about safety and cannot find the information you need, protect your child's health by consulting with an herbal practitioner.

GROWING YOUR OWN HERBS: HOW TO START

If you have a sunny window, a balcony, or a yard, you can grow herbs. There is nothing like picking your own basil for pesto, snipping a bit of mint for a cup of tea, or even digging up your own horseradish!

If a container garden is necessary due to space restrictions, opt for annual herbs (those that live for only one growing season) and choose the largest container that fits the space. A larger container will accommodate several plants and also help the herbs retain moisture longer, so they survive even if you miss a day of watering.

Now comes the fun part. Decide if the herbs will be culinary, medicinal, or both. Sneak a tomato plant in there, and maybe a pepper or two.

Good culinary choices for beginners are parsley, sage, rosemary, and thyme. Dill is a favorite here, too.

Medicinal herb choices for beginners include holy basil, lemon balm, calendula, mint, and chamomile.

All of these plants can be purchased from your local nurseries, which usually have the best varieties for your region. Grow them as annuals; if they do come back, it's a bonus.

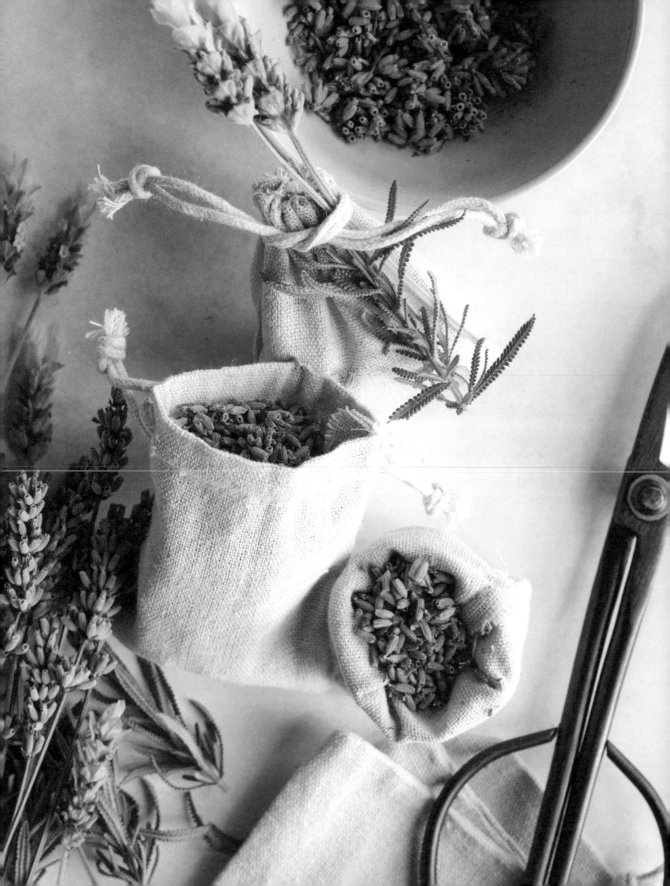

CHAPTER TWO

The Best Herbs for You

When you begin learning about herbs for health, you may try a cup of a certain tea for a particular issue, or maybe some tincture for a different problem, without considering whether it is truly your best choice. The more you learn, the more you'll find that you can match specific herbs to different types of people and their conditions in order to have a more effective result.

In Western herbalism, this concept is called herbal energetics, and many people find that it helps them understand how to choose remedies more easily. This is explained in more detail in this chapter.

Energetics of Individuals

Most cultures have a healing tradition that helps make the connection between a person's constitution and what kind of herbs will help bring them back to balance. Examples from around the world include Ayurveda, traditional Chinese medicine, the Indigenous Medicine Wheel, and Southern folk herbalism. These traditions are all essentially different forms of energetics. In this chapter, we'll examine the philosophy of traditional Western medicine energetics, which is more than 100 years old and a melding of many traditions.

Individual energetics refers to one's constitution, which is the general condition of the body. It is important to choose the right herb energy for the constitution of the person. Determine your own constitution by pondering the following list. For some people, it will be as clear as a bell, but for others it may require some examination and thought.

My own constitution is damp and neutral temperature (neither hot nor cold), tending toward lax.

Some of the things that lead me to this classification are my ability to sweat on cue and the feeling that it might be possible to die from humidity (damp). I have many hot and cold markers, so that lands me in the neutral territory. If nobody forces me to move around and do things, I'll probably take a couple naps and not get dressed for the day (lax).

HERE ARE THE TYPES:

Cool/cold:

- Cold hands and feet
- Pale complexion
- Quiet
- Sluggish or inactive
- Would like another sweater, please

Damp:

- Ankles may swell easily
- Does not like humidity
- Oily skin and hair
- Prone to congestion or runny nose
- Retains water easily
- Sweats easily and freely

Dry:

- Brittle nails, hair breaks easily
- Creaky joints
- Dry skin and scalp
- Itchy
- Prone to constipation
- Prone to dry cough and throat

Lax/relaxed:

- At its worst, may mean loss of muscle control
- Prone to depression (physical and emotional)
- Sleepy, difficult to wake
- Sluggish, stagnant

Tense:

- Headaches
- Nervous or irritable, easily rattled
- Tight, painful muscles
- Too busy

Warm/hot:

- Always doing something active, can be hyper
- Blushes easily
- Healthy appetite
- Outspoken
- Usually feels warm

We all land somewhere between hot and cold, damp and dry, tense and lax. Those things all change from time to time, but we tend toward one side or the other unless drastic life changes occur. For instance, I have seen a warm, damp person become cool and dry after chemotherapy.

If neither type in one category applies, or if they seem equal, you may have a neutral, or balanced, constitution, and that's a good thing. Balance is the goal in health, as it is in all things. Your constitution is part of who you are through heredity and ethnicity, so you can't change it completely, but you can make changes through herbs, food, and lifestyle that move you toward balance.

Personally, I notice that weight changes, age, activity level, and eating habits alter my constitution. Weight gain can bring lots of water retention and bogginess to my body, causing me to perspire more often and lean toward the damp type. Losing weight and upping activity, along with eating lots of good fresh fruits and vegetables, can return me to a more balanced constitution with more control of moisture, tone, and temperature. Similarly, someone with a cold, dry constitution can sometimes neutralize that with hydration, exercise (to warm the muscles and organs), and consumption of warming, moist foods.

For home herbalists, knowing your baseline constitution is valuable. It helps you understand the foods and herbs that can steer you closer to the center, as well as the foods and herbs that you want to avoid. Understanding your own constitution and that of those close to you enables you to choose the correct herb for the individual.

Energetics of Herbs

Now that you understand the types of constitution/tissue states, you can select herbs that correspond to each one. Yes, herbs have energetics, too! The trick is to work with herbs that promote balance in the body. For instance, a cooling herb would be called for in a hot state, a drying herb would be called for in a damp state, and a relaxing herb would be called for in a tense state. Here are some common examples:

COOLING hibiscus, lavender, lettuce, raspberry leaf, watermelon

DRYING goldenrod, osha, sage, tea, turmeric, yarrow

MOISTURIZING licorice, marshmallow root, okra, plantain, purslane, slippery elm

RELAXING catnip, chamomile, hops, lavender, lemon balm, valerian

TONING (INVIGORATES TONE AND TIGHTNESS) blackberry leaf, lady's mantle, rose, tea, witch hazel, yarrow

WARMING basil, black pepper, cayenne, cinnamon, garlic, ginger

Within the various types, many herbs have different actions. For instance, when it comes to relaxing herbs, chamomile very gently calms anxiety, milky oat seed supports the nervous system, passionflower helps with circular thinking that creates tension, and skullcap relieves stress and mental exhaustion. Herbs work in different and powerful ways.

Furthermore, the tastes of herbs and foods also correspond to the energetics of herbs. The taste of an herb reinforces its action. Here are the tastes most often used in herbal healing, with some examples:

ASTRINGENT (DRY) cranberries, oregano, parsley, tea

BITTER (COLD, DAMP) citrus peel, dandelion, gentian, hops, mugwort, yellow dock

PUNGENT (HOT, DRY) cumin, horseradish, mustard, paprika

SALTY (COLD, DRY) celery, nettles, seaweed, soy sauce, vinegar

SOUR (COOL, DRY) fermented foods, lemon, sumac, tamarind

SPICY (WARM, DRY) cinnamon, cloves, ginger, holy basil

SWEET (WARM, DAMP) anise, cardamom, nutmeg, sesame seeds

When choosing herbs, keep in mind that the goal is always to move from an excess of a particular constitutional element toward balance. If an illness exhibits cold and wet symptoms, you want to respond with herbs that are warm/hot and dry to balance them out.

Let's say someone is hot, dry, and tense in constitution, and this is causing issues with constipation. You'd want to choose cooling, demulcent, or moistening herbs that tend to have a sweet taste. Licorice root, slippery elm, and marshmallow root would all be helpful for this person.

If we combine the herbs that will work in balance with the person's constitution and the tastes that affect that action, we can be better assured that we're choosing the correct herb for the situation.

Energetics of Illnesses

Many years ago, my sister and I were on a road trip and chatting about how difficult it is to accurately describe pain to the doctor. At some point she said hers was a round, sweet pain. We laughed for about 10 miles after that one.

Looking back, I see that we were onto something, but we just weren't using the terminology of a recognized tradition. The truth is that illnesses have energetics, too.

Once you become familiar with the energetics of humans and herbs, it becomes clear how they correlate to the symptoms of an illness and how best to approach and treat that illness. One way to look at it is that the illness presents itself by demonstrating in what way the body is out of balance. Heat needs to be cooled; damp requires drying. Simple yet true.

Consider the language we use to describe an illness or its symptoms. How often do we use the terms that describe the tissue states, or variations of the terms? "This cold is stuck in my chest," or "My back is so tense that it's got my head aching, too." It's already how we think about illness. Now we just need to put it all together.

Let's say your child has a weeping skin rash (damp). Your goal will be to dry it up so it can heal. You wouldn't put oil or any kind of barrier over it, because it needs contact with the air to dry. If you had dry, painful patches such as brush burns or cracked hands, you wouldn't reach for a drying treatment like a drawing clay poultice. You likely know all this instinctively, without having to think about the energetics involved.

Eventually, this system of healing becomes second nature. I encourage people to think about how much they use this system without realizing it, then go from there. It is important to learn which actions each herb has and how it works.

Another thing to consider is whether herbs are associated with a certain organ or body part. This will narrow down your possible choices when approaching an illness or ailment. Here are just a few examples:

GOLDENROD kidney

HAWTHORN AND ROSE heart

MILK THISTLE liver

OATS nervous system

PLEURISY ROOT lining of lungs and chest cavity

SOLOMON'S SEAL connective tissues

If you struggle to classify some herbs, tissues, and illnesses into types and states, that's okay. Even experts don't always agree. As Rosemary Gladstar once told a class I attended, "Put three herbalists in a room, and you'll get three different opinions." The main thing is to trust your knowledge and intuition.

The next chapter will give you a lot of tools for your herbal toolkit. It will teach you how to make various herbal concoctions and give you an idea of how everything works together. Then that will just leave the herbs.

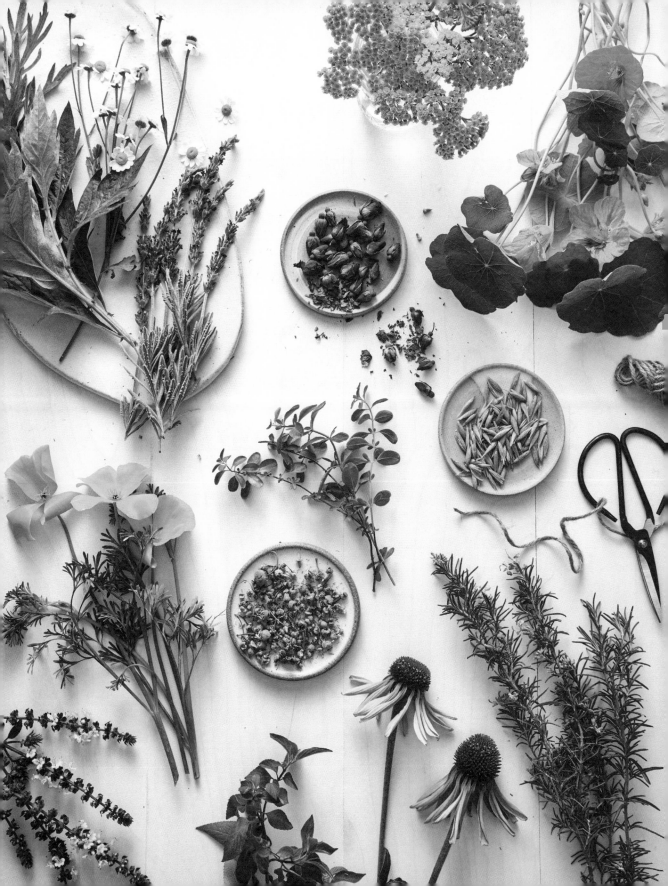

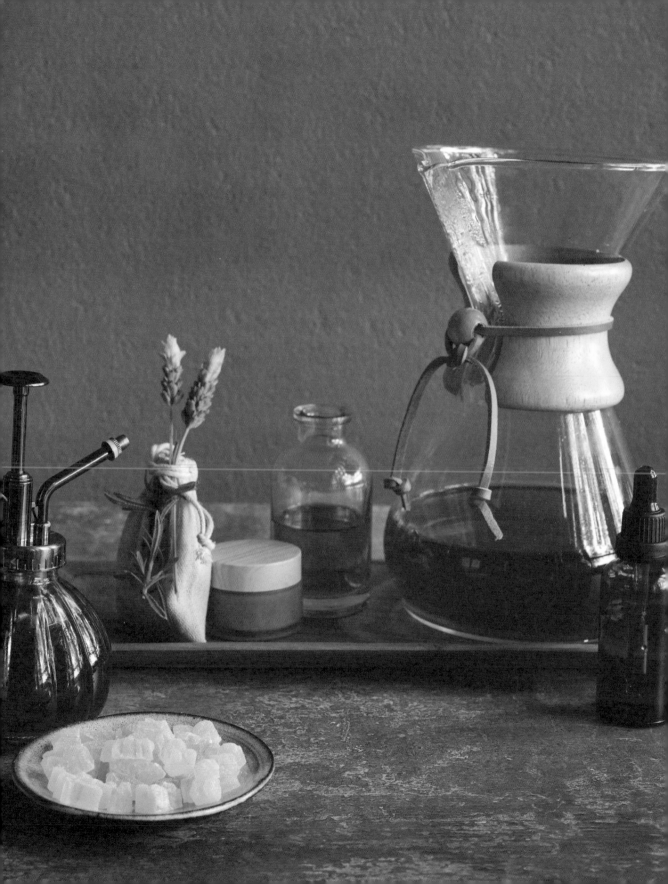

CHAPTER THREE

Getting Started with Herbal Medicine

The exciting part of your journey with herbs is learning all the ways you can bring herbs into your life. The act of harvesting chamomile, calendula, or rose petals is, in itself, healing, which may explain why so many of us enjoy bringing plants and flowers into our homes.

Finding out how to easily and inexpensively create a vast array of remedies, formulations, and concoctions is life changing. How wonderful to learn how to make a bath into a spa! Imagine knowing how to pluck a few leaves, roots, or berries and create remedies for hundreds of discomforts or illnesses.

It all starts with learning how to create your own apothecary.

What You'll Need

It's time for the fun part! This chapter covers nine herbal preparations, and you'll need a few supplies at the ready. Don't worry, you don't need anything fancy—my guess is that you have most of these items in your kitchen already. Anything else can easily be found at a craft or kitchen supply store (or even the dollar store). I also offer DIY alternatives wherever possible.

First things first: Start saving every jar you use! Grab them back out of the recycling bin, wash them, and save them. The same goes for any smallish plastic container that seals, as well as clean zip-top bags.

SUPPLIES:

- Cutting board

- Double boiler

- Dropper bottles

- Filters (DIY: clean, old T-shirts cut into 6-by-6-inch squares)

- Funnels in various sizes (DIY: Cut off the top half of a used plastic bottle. These make great funnels and can be used over and over.)

- Jars in varying sizes

- Knife (a good sharp one)

- Labels (big enough to write on)

- Measuring cups

- Measuring spoons

- Muslin bags for compresses (DIY: material from clean, old cotton or flannel sheets)

- Scale. If you find that you really enjoy making salves and balms and want to make any quantity, the ingredients should be weighed. A decent scale is always a good investment.

- Strainers, both fine and regular mesh

- Tea infusers (or tea balls), one small (for individual cups) and one large (for pots of tea). The perforated metal balls are most common, but you can also find these made of silicone in different, fun shapes, as well as other types of infusers.

- Non-herbal ingredients:

- Alcohol, typically vodka (190-proof is excellent, 151-proof is the next choice, and 100-proof also works)

- Beeswax (sold in craft stores and health-food stores)

- Olive oil

These are the basic supplies you need to get started. When we get to the individual sections, I suggest additional options, but you can generally make do without those. After a little practice, you can also come up with your own way of doing things—that's part of the fun.

For many years, these were the only tools I used. As time went by, I acquired a distiller to make hydrosols and essential oils, a press specifically made to extract all the oil or liquid from an infusion, and a couple food processors. I love them, but I managed for a long time without them.

Two other things you'll need are time and space. Keep in mind that these are healing preparations, and therefore you want to pay attention to your intentions and your mood while creating them. Try to pour some love and care into these concoctions as you work. Clear a space. Put on some good music. Take your time and enjoy the process. Certainly, that isn't always possible. Sometimes the kid is in the bedroom hacking away, you're tired, and there's a bit of vomit streaked down your back. Of course, you'll do what you need to do depending on the situation.

But if you can carve out some dedicated time to prepare an herbal medicine arsenal that's ready and waiting for the next cold, flu, or upset stomach, it's worth it. The first time someone asks for your special tea, or you can produce a healing tincture at the snap of a finger, it's a great feeling.

DOSAGE

The vast majority of herbs, when used with a little knowledge, are gentle and don't require dosages as precise as medicinal drugs. The dosage generally depends on the herb, the individual, the energetics (covered in the next chapter), and the issue or ailment being addressed.

When using a new herb, the best thing to do is start with a small amount. If it's a tea, start with a cup and see how you feel. With a tincture, 12 to 15 drops is a good start. For syrup, a teaspoon or two will do. On the rare occasions when I get sick, these rules go out the window because after years of trial and error, I know how different herbs affect me. You may find me wandering around with a box of tissues, swigging from a bottle of elderberry syrup or pouring it into my giant mug of ginger, honey, and lemon tea. Over time, I've gained a deep understanding of what works for me.

Taking too much of an herb can result in minor diarrhea (similar to eating too much broccoli or cabbage), sleeplessness or sleepiness, or something similarly benign. If you don't experience these symptoms, feel free to slowly increase your dose if desired.

To determine a child's dosage, consider their weight. We generally assume an average adult weight to be about 150 pounds. If the adult dose is 30 drops, then a 30-pound child would get one-fifth of the adult dose, or 6 drops. Another helpful trick is using one drop per year of age up to age 12. As mentioned previously, herbs are not as exacting as pharmaceutical drugs, but it's always smart to err on the side of caution when it comes to children.

Specific dosage guidelines are difficult to find. You can consult with an herbalist if you're feeling unsure and looking for more guidance. And always speak with an herbalist or doctor when working with a chronic condition or illness.

LABELING

Always label your preparations! Do this as soon as you're done making them. Skipping this step is how I ended up with my famous shelf of unknown remedies. There are still times when I'll be called away in the middle of preparing something and forget to label what I added, and the memory instantly fades. The second there's even a fleeting doubt, it's too late, and you can't be certain what went into your preparation.

Your labels should include:

NAME OF THE REMEDY

INGREDIENTS

DATE MADE

INSTRUCTIONS FOR USE

Start a notebook from the moment you begin creating formulas. Write down the steps as you work so you know how to re-create things. There's nothing worse than making the world's best-ever tea blend and then forgetting what went into it.

If stored in the refrigerator, most preparations can last between six months and a year. Without preservatives, that's a good rule of thumb.

STORAGE

When it comes to storing herbal preparations, first and foremost, date your jars! Since they are not chemically preserved, you want to throw them out after a year (unless they are obviously past their prime before then). Tinctures are an exception and can last for up to 10 years if properly stored, but a year is a good guideline for most everything else. Here are some storage tips:

- Use bottles or jars that have a dark color, such as amber or blue. This goes for dried herbs as well.

- Store in a cool, dry place. If the remedy is used in the bathroom, keep just a small container there and store the rest either in the refrigerator or in a cupboard.

- Freezing or refrigeration will extend the life of oils and syrups.

Herbal Teas

Herbal teas are one of the easiest and most pleasant ways to incorporate herbs into your daily life. Sometimes teas are called tisanes; when only a single herb is used for a tea, it is called a simple tea. But most people just call them herbal teas.

Herbal teas are differentiated from the teas made from the plant *Camellia sinensis*, which include black, green, oolong, and white teas. These all come from a single plant, which is technically an herb that contains caffeine! What we consider to be herbal teas do not have caffeine, so that's the main distinction.

Lots of people are only vaguely aware of the medicinal properties of the teas that they've come to regularly enjoy. Herbal teas are one of the gentlest means of taking medicinal herbs. Many of them can be given to children—my daughter still remembers the chamomile tea parties we'd have during scary thunderstorms or other stressful times. Twenty-plus years later, chamomile is still a favorite simple tea that's always in her cupboard.

Teas were my gateway herbs. After spending a winter reading various herb books, I spent the spring, summer, and fall gathering sprigs and petals of every possible herb I could use for tea, pinching bits from gardens of friends or running across a meadow for something. I dried them on a screen and mixed them together in a big jar. I added some purchased stevia leaves, cinnamon chips (chopped dried cinnamon bark), and licorice root, and shook it up. We brewed the concoction by the cup. Each cup was different, and there wasn't a bad one in the bunch.

There are a couple of different brewing methods. When using the more tender parts of the plant, like the leaves, the herbs are infused. This involves pouring hot water over the herbs (which you can place in a tea ball or tea bag) and letting them steep for 5 to 15 minutes before straining.

Don't confuse this technique with the recent popularity of the word *infusion*, as in "herbal infusions." This refers to a very concentrated beverage made using one ounce of dried herb in a quart of water and steeping overnight. There are only a handful of plants suited to this method, including vitamin- and mineral-laden herbs like stinging nettle, red clover, and oats.

As a general guideline, use a teaspoon of dried herb or herb blend or a tablespoon of fresh herbs per one cup (8 ounces) of tea. That said, the measurement isn't critical with tea. I usually go over because I keep adding things!

Teas made with denser bark, seeds, or roots are decocted. I'll often make up a decoction of wild cherry bark, licorice root, fennel seeds, and perhaps a couple of other roots, depending on the purpose. To decoct, simmer the herb in water for an extended period, which can be from 15 minutes to several hours depending on the herb. The harder the material, the more heat and time that are needed to extract the properties and flavors.

In terms of which herbs to use for your teas, a lot depends on where you live and what is available. Some good herbs to try are mint, chamomile, sage, thyme, hibiscus, jasmine, passionflower, or lemon balm. Sprinkle in some rose petals. Raspberry and blueberry leaves add flavor and have useful components.

For a simple, relaxing tea, try blending chamomile, passionflower, and lemon balm.

To soothe a cold and sore throat, try sage, thyme, and elder with a licorice root stir stick.

Upset stomach? Ginger tea with a little spearmint can work wonders.

Teas are especially valuable for comfort and calming.

Syrups

Making syrups is a simple way to preserve herbs using inexpensive ingredients. Some syrups are tasty enough to drizzle over ice cream or crepes, or into cock-tails or shrubs. Syrups can take the most horrendous flavor and make it palatable enough for a child to enjoy. Horehound is a good example: It's an acquired taste, at best (although there are people who like it), but it's terrific for soothing coughs and a variety of upper-respiratory issues. Mixing it with some sugar, honey, or molasses helps the medicine go right down.

To make syrup, you'll need a pan, strainer, measuring cups, funnel, bottles, and a spoon.

Start with a strong herbal tea that has been simmered down to reduce by about half. Next, add either 2 parts sugar (1 cup of tea, 2 cups of sugar) or an equal amount of honey or molasses (1 cup of tea, 1 cup of honey or molasses). I generally use sugar because it's inexpensive and I always have it in the house. Stir to be sure the sugar (or honey or molasses) is dissolved, bring to a rolling boil, and continue to boil for about 3 minutes. Cool, bottle, cap, and label.

Syrups can keep for up to a year in the refrigerator. If you want to store without refrigeration, concentrate the infusion more by simmering it down to about one-third the original quantity, and add 1/4 cup of 100-proof vodka for every 1 cup of syrup (resulting in 12.5 percent alcohol content).

This alcohol content is not much when taken by the teaspoon, but be aware of it for children and people who are or might be pregnant.

Elderberry syrup (pages 162 and 181) is a must-have every year for winter health. This staple syrup in our household is one that's great for soothing mucus in the throat and chest.

A simple ginger syrup is good to have around because once it's in the cabinet, you'll be reaching for it to add to teas, baked goods, stir-fries, and so much more. Blackstrap molasses makes a tasty and nourishing base.

In the spring, violet, rose, and dandelion syrups are fun and beautiful to make. Those herbs work best with a sugar base and some lemon, which allow the gorgeous colors to come through.

Oils

Infused herbal oils are made by soaking herbs in a vegetable or nut oil for an extended period, with or without heat. It is important to mention that this is completely different from an essential oil.

Many different oils can be infused. Olive is the most common because it's easy to find, affordable, and great for the skin. Sweet almond oil is often found as an ingredient in older herbals, but it tends to go rancid quickly if not refrigerated. Apricot, avocado, sesame, hazelnut, sunflower, and jojoba (technically a wax, making it extremely shelf stable) oils are also good options.

Most herbal oil infusions are used topically in salves, balms, lotions, soaps, and massage oils. They can be used as culinary oils, but that requires extreme caution, as any moisture at all can result in botulism.

There are several methods for making herbal oils. The key is to make sure that no water is introduced into the oil. The moisture that is in the plant material must be allowed to evaporate freely or the oil will develop mold. Additionally, all plant material must be completely covered by oil to avoid mold.

To make infused oil, you'll need a large glass measuring cup, a strainer, a jar for storing, and, if using fresh herbs, cheesecloth.

The easiest method is to start with dried herbs in oil using gentle heat. The oven on the lowest setting or a slow cooker equipped with a low setting works very well, and a jar of oil and herbs sitting in a south-facing window is great. I'm always in a hurry, so it's the slow cooker overnight for me. The oven would also be overnight, and the window could take a few weeks.

If you want to use fresh herbs, which can be tricky, they should be well wilted to lessen their water content. After mixing the herbs into the oil, cover the jar with several layers of cheesecloth to allow evaporation until the infusion is finished. The infusion is done when it has taken on the scent and/or color of the herb, usually after at least two weeks. (Many years ago, I made a gallon of jewelweed oil and didn't wilt the herb or allow it to evaporate, keeping the bottle sealed. It looked great, but when I opened the jug in the spring, the oil was putrid.)

When the oil is finished, strain out the herbs. I have a favorite method for straining: using 6-inch squares of material from old T-shirts. Line a mesh strainer with one of these squares and set it over a large (2-quart) glass measuring cup. Then, pour the oil and herbs slowly through it. Squeeze the material to get all the good oil into the cup. Pour the oil into a jar or bottle, screw on the top, and label it.

You can also infuse solid oils like shea, coconut, cocoa butter, soy, and mango butter. Liquefy them with gentle heat and then introduce the herbs. On warm, sunny days, you can put them in the heat of the sun until they are liquid and then add your herbs. After several hours, put the oil in the refrigerator and keep it there until you need it. At that time, heat the oil to liquid again, strain out the plant material, and use the oil.

In the following sections, you'll see how you can mix oils into a variety of preparations like salves, balms, and massage oils to add a healing herbal component.

Salves

Salves are emollient and healing blends of herbal oils. You can make all-purpose salves for any skin problem, antiseptic salves for healing wounds; drawing salves for pulling out splinters, venom, and infections; salves for chest rubs; or salves for sore muscles. They can even be made as a pleasant hand softener or lip balm. Salves, lip balms, and the more solid lotion bar are all basically the same thing. The only difference is the amount of beeswax used. Once you learn this skill, it comes in handy for all sorts of things—salve variations can be used for hair pomade, diaper rash cream, and even furniture polish!

To add herbs to salves, the herbs are first infused in oil, then blended with beeswax. Vegan options for wax include bayberry, candelilla, or cocoa butter.

Here are some general starting points:

SALVE 1 part wax to 8 parts oil

LIP BALM 1 part wax to 4 parts oil

LOTION BARS 1 part wax to 2 parts oil

To make a salve, you'll need a double boiler (or a microwave and glass measuring cup), a stainless-steel spoon, jars, and labels.

Start with about one-fourth of the oil to be used and mix it with the wax. Heat the mixture to melt the wax. You can do this in either a double boiler or the microwave. If using the microwave, heat in 30-second increments, stirring after each. Either way, continue until the wax is completely melted. Be sure the remaining oil is at room temperature, then add it to the wax mixture. This prevents heating all of the oil to the melting point of the wax. But don't worry, you can't really ruin a salve. You simply add more oil or more wax until you have the right consistency.

Tinctures

Tinctures may sound scientific and intimidating, but as it turns out, this folk method couldn't be easier. Tinctures are simply plants steeped in alcohol for a period of time until the liquid becomes much like a very concentrated tea. Fresh herbal properties can be well preserved in a tincture with almost no work and just a little time.

I always keep chamomile tincture around. My daughter was anxious as a child and had difficulty falling asleep, and I found that chamomile was just the thing to help her. I also keep a blend of holy basil and mimosa flower on hand for emotionally draining situations when I can't see the forest for the trees.

You'll need a knife or scissors, a cutting board, alcohol (typically vodka), jars, and labels. Wilt the herbs to get rid of excess moisture, and then use a good-quality vodka (150-proof is my go-to). Some people prefer whiskey, rum, or brandy; it's just a matter of taste. Fill a jar with chopped herbs. Cover with your alcohol of choice. Leave at room temperature for six weeks, shaking the jar daily (or when you remember). After six weeks, strain the mixture and your tincture is ready for use.

Some people put their herbs in a food processor first. Some people shake their jars every day. If you don't need to use the tincture right away, you can leave it unstrained for years. Tinctures can keep for many years whether strained or with the herbs left in the alcohol.

To use a tincture, start at a low dose and see how it works. Mix it with a swallow of water or juice. Tinctures don't always taste great, so get it over with quickly. Some people choose to put tinctures straight under their tongues, but in my opinion, there's no need to suffer like that. You can also mix a dose into a cup of tea (even herbal tea) or juice.

Regarding the alcohol in tinctures: The typical dosage is less than a teaspoon of alcohol. Most sources will say that this is equivalent to the naturally occurring alcohol content in a ripe banana. I never hesitated to give a few drops mixed in juice to my toddler. As long as the herb is safe to use during pregnancy, this amount of alcohol shouldn't be a problem. Still, I would never suggest that someone who cannot have alcohol should use tinctures. There are lots of other good ways to ingest herbs, so why risk it?

If alcohol isn't an option for you for whatever reason, you can substitute glycerin, using 3 parts glycerin to 1 part water. However, the tinctures last for only about a year using this method.

Pills

Pills (or pastilles) are another remedy that is very easy and inexpensive to make. There's nothing in the pills except the herb and whatever liquid or moistener is used to form the pill. You can use any herb or combination of herbs, and, with practice, the pills can be made to be quite tasty. I particularly like to use them for sore throats.

To make pills, combine freshly powdered herbs with a liquid to form a thick, firm paste.* The paste is then rolled into balls, which may or may not be flattened into a lozenge shape, and then dried. These come in handy for children—the pills can be made smaller or larger, depending on what the child can hold in their mouth and how much herb is desired. To take the pill, hold it in your mouth until it breaks apart and can be swallowed.

You'll need a bowl, knife, spoon, jars or tins, and labels. It's very important to finely powder the herbs. I like to use a coffee grinder and then put the powder through a mesh strainer to remove any larger bits. You can also purchase powdered herbs, but be aware that powders lose their vitality very quickly. It's always best to keep herbs as whole as possible until use.

Next, choose your liquid. Honey is typically my first choice, but you can also use tea, glycerin, coconut oil, or a medicinal syrup you've made. Start with 2 parts herbal powder to 1 part liquid. Add the liquid a bit at a time, and knead the mixture very well, adding more liquid as needed. Get similar-size pieces by rolling the "dough" into a log and cutting off short lengths. Dry thoroughly. Dry pills should be shelf stable for several months, but I stick them in the refrigerator or freezer out of habit. They'll basically last forever if frozen.

The mixture before drying is called an electuary, which can be added to or used to make herbal teas.

Another easy way to make a pill is to get empty capsules and fill them with powdered herbs. These are meant to be swallowed and are sometimes the only way to get someone to take a bitter herb!

Baths

Herbs in the tub can do a lot. As a child, I remember my mother putting me in the kitchen sink full of oatmeal water, probably for the measles or chicken pox. It was so soothing. A cup of vinegar steeped with roses poured into a tepid bath is a wonder for sunburn. Comfrey and Epsom salts after too much physical activity relax muscles and help achy joints. The list goes on and on. A nice herbal bath can be so healing.

Baths are very similar to teas in the way they are made. You can often drink the same product created for bathing, and honey can even be part of the deal.

I prefer to fill a half-gallon pitcher with very hot water, then submerge a muslin bag filled with the herbs in the water while running a bath. It makes a strong "tea" that you can then pour into the bath. No muslin bag? No worries. Place the herbs in the center of a washcloth, bind the corners with a rubber band, and make your "tea" that way.

You can put additions like oatmeal, powdered milk, or salt in the bag or directly into the bath water. Just be careful not to clog the drain.

Herbs for the bath can be used in fresh or dried forms. Good choices are comfrey root and leaf, calendula flowers, roses, lavender, chamomile, mint, yarrow, plantain leaf, jewelweed, rosemary, thyme, elderflower, chickweed, seaweed, and sage.

Poultices

Poultices are used to treat issues by applying herbs directly to the skin. They are typically, but not always, used for external issues. They may be used to soothe or calm rashes, and are also valuable for drawing out toxins, stings, and splinters. Making herbal poultices can be as simple as chewing up a leaf and putting the wet, mashed herb onto an insect bite or wound. Or, it can be as involved as heating a mixture of herbs in oil and applying it to the skin, covered with layers of material.

Tea bag poultices are easy and quick, and people commonly use them without thinking of them as poultices. For instance, years ago it felt like I might be developing a stye on my eye, so I brewed up two tea bags in one cup, one chamomile and one echinacea, to put on the affected eye. As one tea bag cooled, I would replace it on my eye with the other. Rotating the tea bags stopped the stye or infection from getting a foothold.

"Spit poultices" are hurried preparations made in the field. For example, for yellow jacket or wasp stings, an instant remedy is a plantain leaf chewed and applied to the sting after removing the stinger. It provides immediate relief, and if done promptly, draws out the venom before damage occurs.

I once had a blocked salivary gland. After spending a good deal of time finding the gland, I made small, half-moon-shaped poultices in heat-sealable tea bags. I filled them with a blend of plantain, chickweed, and kaolin clay, and they successfully pulled the little "stone" out.

A mustard plaster placed on the chest would be considered a poultice, as would the old-time practice of chopping and cooking large amounts of onions and spreading them as hot as could be borne on the chest. Both of these treatments have a layer of cloth between them and the skin to prevent skin irritation. They're both commonly used to increase circulation and loosen chest congestion.

Compresses

Most everyone has used a hot or cold compress after a muscle injury. Herbal compresses are similar but have the added healing properties of herbs. Compresses can be prepared for use at different temperatures, depending on the purpose. Hot compresses are used for muscular pains, cramping, and drawing out infections. Most other issues call for room-temperature or cool compresses.

Making a compress is very easy: For smaller areas, grab a thick washcloth, or use a hand towel for larger areas. Make a very strong herbal tea in a quantity that will allow you to saturate the cloth, then soak the cloth in the tea and wring it out. Place the soaked cloth on the affected area for 15 to 30 minutes, repeating as needed.

If you prefer a cold compress, place the soaked cloth in the freezer briefly (take it out before it freezes). This is faster than waiting for the tea to cool down. Teas brewed for compresses can be refrigerated or frozen and reheated when needed. Be sure to label any frozen teas like you would other preparations. It's no fun to find containers of herbal ice cubes and have no clue as to what they might contain.

Here are some of my go-to compresses:

ACHING OR NERVE PAIN Lemon balm with St. John's wort, used either very warm or very cold, perhaps alternating.

ECZEMA Plantain, chickweed, calendula, and lavender applied at room temperature.

GENERAL RASH Chamomile, applied cool or at room temperature to soothe and calm the skin.

MUSCLE SPRAINS OR STRAINS WITH NO BROKEN SKIN Arnica with comfrey and Epsom salts, applied warm.

PLANT RASHES (POISON IVY, OAK, SUMAC) Yarrow with jewelweed and plantain applied as a cool compress.

SUNBURN Black tea with lavender and rose petals. This should be used as a cool, but not cold, compress.

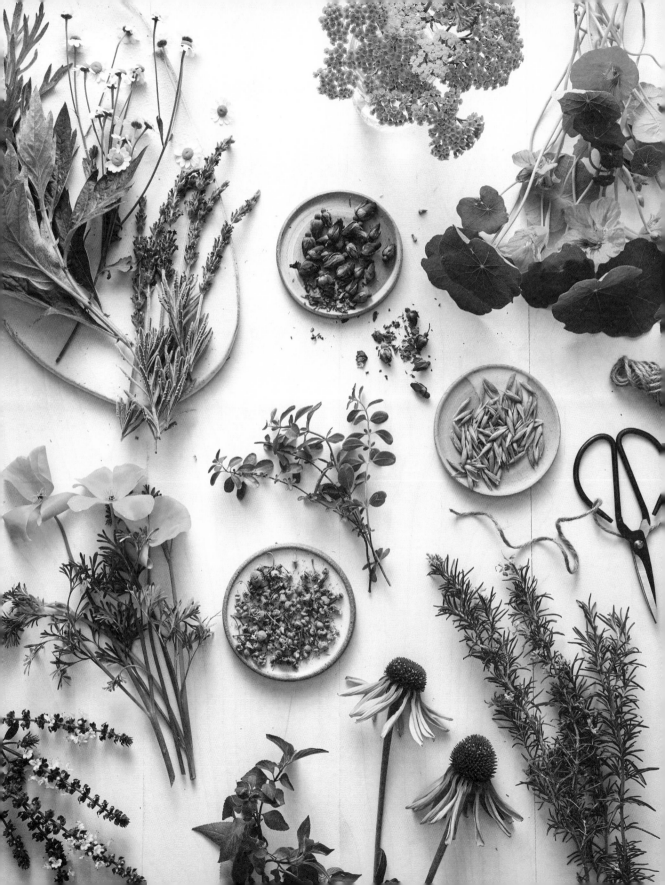

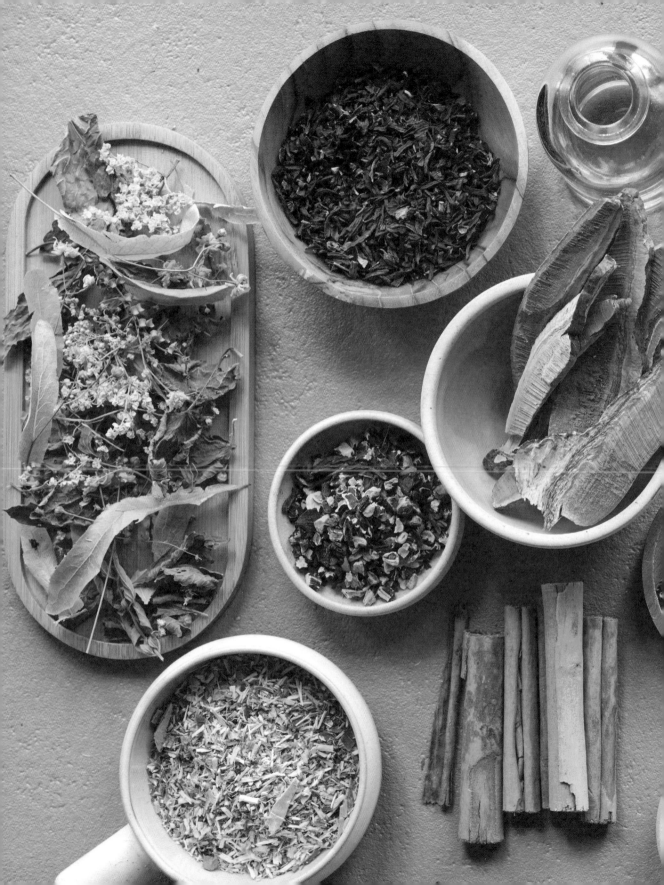

PART TWO

Herbs for Healing

One of the most intimidating things about herbalism is the sheer number of possibilities. "How will I ever know all of these plants?"

Honestly, nobody knows them all. Dr. James Duke traveled to the rain forests looking for new (to him) plants, and Chris Kilham, aka "The Medicine Hunter," goes all over the world finding a seemingly never-ending array of plants. There are herbs out there that humans will never even discover.

The good news is that you don't need to know all of them. This section provides detailed information for 90 different herbs, which is more than enough to get you started.

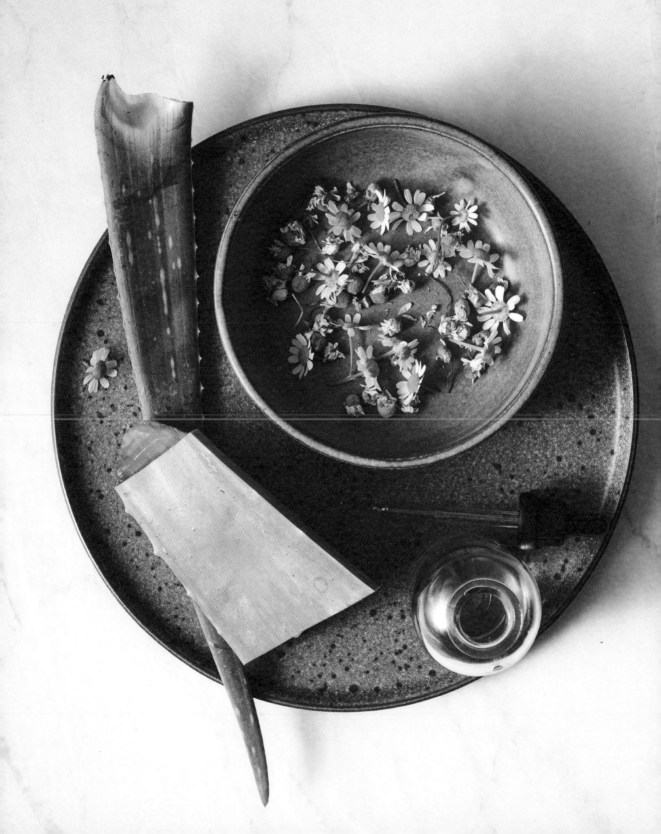

CHAPTER FOUR

Nature's Apothecary

This chapter contains information on a wide variety of herbs, all with amazing abilities and offerings. It is incredibly comforting to walk into the kitchen, put on the teakettle, and blend up a tea for a son with indigestion, a daughter with cramps, or an elder who can't sleep. Opening a cupboard to find syrups, vinegars, and tonics when a virus is about is immensely comforting. The herbs that follow are all relatively easy to obtain. They are safe (except in the circumstances noted), and most are stunningly versatile. For each herb listed here, you'll find the best way to prepare and use it as well as any necessary warnings.

Aloe

Latin Name: *Aloe barbadensis*
Common Name(s): Burn plant, medicine plant, plant of immortality, sinkle bible (particularly in the Caribbean Islands)

Vital Parts:

The gel and firm pulp (also known as the fillet, or tuna) inside the leaves; the bitter yellow latex, called aloe juice, or sap that forms between the green skin and the clear gel in mature plants.

Medicinal Uses:

Externally, aloe can heal wounds, burns, skin infections, psoriasis, and eczema. One of its natural constituents is salicylic acid, which helps promote skin turnover. It also contains vitamins A, C, and E to help nourish the skin. Internally, it's good for digestive issues such as irritable bowel syndrome (IBS), constipation, and ulcers.

Safety Considerations:

Regular and long-term internal use of aloe can cause chronic diarrhea and at high doses may cause liver damage, so it is strongly discouraged beyond occasional use. Aloe should not be used internally during pregnancy or while breastfeeding. If you use insulin or blood thinners or have hypoglycemia, do not take aloe internally. Some individuals may be allergic to it.

Preparations:

Capsules, creams, gels, juices, lotions, soaps

TIP: The only way to kill aloe is to overwater it, so let it dry out. Cut the leaves from the bottom to use, as they'll be the oldest and largest. Aloe grows as a perennial in zones 9 and 10, with lance-shaped leaves from the basal rosette reaching several feet tall.

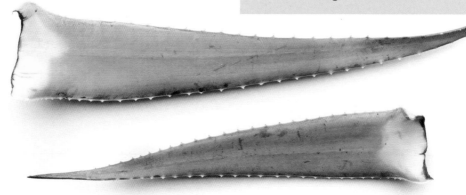

Arnica

Latin Name: *Arnica montana*
Common Name(s): Leopard's bane, mountain tobacco, wolf's bane

Vital Parts:
Buds, flowers, and leaves

Medicinal Uses:
Arnica is widely used for reducing muscle and joint pain and the swelling and inflammation that often accompany these conditions. Similarly, it can be used to treat osteoarthritis, bruises, and insect bites. Arnica is also commonly used to treat dandruff, strengthen hair, and promote hair growth. It also nourishes chapped lips.

Safety Considerations:
Herbal medicines made with arnica are for external use only. If taken internally, there is potential for heart arrhythmias and respiratory failure. If you develop a rash associated with topical arnica use, wash the affected area thoroughly with soap and water and discontinue use.

Preparations:
gels, hair tonics, lip balms, oils, ointments, poultices, sprays, topical

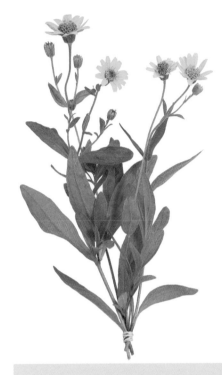

TIP: There are many excellent arnica products available at major retailers, health-food stores, and from online retailers. Arnica can be grown in gardens throughout the Northern Hemisphere. The plants prefer well-drained soil and tend to thrive when a bit of gravel is added to the growing medium. Propagation is best achieved by root division early in the growing season, but seeds may be planted as well. Harvest the aerial parts when they are in full bloom.

Ashwagandha

Latin Name: *Withania somnifera*
Common Name(s): Indian ginseng, poison gooseberry, winter cherry

Vital Parts:
Roots, leaves, flowers, and seeds

Medicinal Uses:
Ashwagandha is an ancient herb, long used in Ayurvedic medicine, which is ideal for addressing emotional and energy issues such as anxiety, stress, depression, and fatigue. It can also help with flagging libido, sleep issues, brain fog, and general debility. Ashwagandha also rejuvenates the skin and helps treat skin issues.

Safety Considerations:
Not for use during pregnancy. If you are taking blood pressure, blood sugar, thyroid, or autoimmune medications, check with your physician before using ashwagandha.

Preparations:
Capsules (roots), poultices (leaves), powdered, tinctures. The powdered root is traditionally blended with honey and/or ghee (clarified butter) to form a thick paste that is taken a spoonful at a time. This paste can be mixed with warm milk in the evening to help with restlessness and to promote sleep.

TIP: The recommended dosage for long-term use in capsules is 250 to 500 mg each day. As tinctures, the recommended dosage is 20 to 60 drops up to 3 times per day.

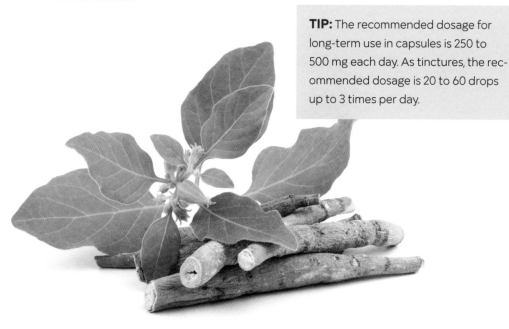

Astragalus

Latin Name: *Astragalus membranaceus*
Common Name(s): Huangqi (China), milk vetch

Vital Parts:
Roots

Medicinal Uses:
Astragalus is often used as a preventive or remedy for upper-respiratory illnesses. It stimulates the immune system and protects the body from the effects of stress. Externally, it soothes and heals the skin. Astragalus is excellent for rebuilding energy and immunity after an illness or when experiencing low energy and strength.

Safety Considerations:
Due to its long history of use, astragalus is generally considered safe, but there have not been enough studies done, so do not use during pregnancy or while breastfeeding. Also avoid astragalus if you're using immunosuppressant medication or have an autoimmune disease.

Preparations:
Capsules, creams, decoctions, lotions, pills, teas, tinctures

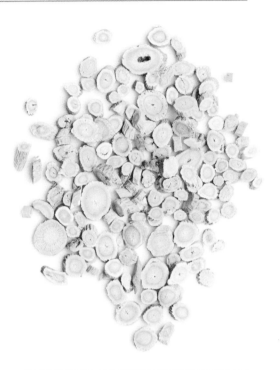

TIP: Astragalus is very easy to grow as a perennial in zones 6 through 9. The vetches can get aggressive, so find a spacious spot where it can spread. You can harvest the roots for use in the fourth year. Dig the outer roots, leaving the center to grow. Clean the roots well, then slice and dry them.

Basil

Latin Name: *Ocimum basilicum*
Common Name(s): Common basil, sweet basil

Vital Parts:
Aerial parts

Medicinal Uses:
Basil is great not only for stimulating the appetite, but also for reducing flatulence and bloated stomach after a meal, as well as treating reactions to gluten and dairy intolerances. It also eases headaches, lowers fevers, combats seasonal affective disorder, clears the mind, lowers blood pressure, calms nervous tension, and clears excess phlegm from the lungs. Basil's distinctive aroma freshens breath while also helping clean the teeth and gums. For nursing mothers, basil increases the flow of milk. You may be surprised to learn that basil is also a wonderful herb to soothe the pain, itch, and inflammation of insect bites and stings, so the next time a friend or family member has an insect bite or sting, reach

for your kitchen basil for relief.

Safety Considerations:
Basil is generally regarded as safe.

Preparations:
Culinary ingredient, teas, tinctures

TIP: Basil is an annual plant that grows to a height of about 2 feet. It prefers full sun, well-drained soil, and a fair amount of water. Fertilize plants with compost at the beginning of the growing season. Pinch back leaves heavily as the plant starts to flower to encourage bushy growth, and harvest as needed.

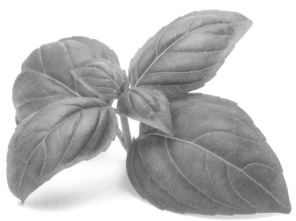

Black Cohosh

Latin Name: *Actaea racemosa*
Common Name(s): Baneberry, black snakeroot, bugbane, phytoestrogen, rattlesnake root, rattleweed, sheng ma, snakeroot

Vital Parts:
Roots or rhizomes

Medicinal Uses:
Anyone with menopause symptoms can benefit from having black cohosh on hand, as it may help treat hot flashes, insomnia, and night sweats. It also suppresses appetite and stimulates metabolism. Black cohosh can also help treat acne, especially in cases caused by hormonal imbalance.

Safety Considerations:
Black cohosh has a similar effect to estrogen, so researchers recommend not taking it if you're breastfeeding, pregnant, diagnosed with breast cancer, or have hormone-sensitive issues that would be triggered by the herb. If you take the herb internally, take a break after one year. Also stop taking it if you're experiencing side effects like upset stomach, headaches, cramps, weight gain, spotting, or bleeding between menstrual periods.

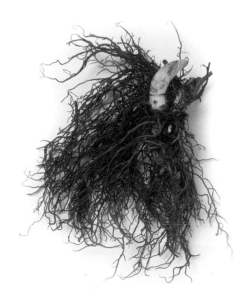

Preparations:
Capsules, standardized extract, teas, tinctures

TIP: Black cohosh plants like to be left in the dark, preferring shade or partial shade over sunlight. They thrive in moist soil and must experience a complete cycle of warm to cold to warm again before the seeds will germinate. Ensure success by planting mature seeds in the fall so they experience the full growth cycle during the plants' first spring.

Black Walnut

Latin Name: *Juglans nigra*
Common Name(s): American walnut, eastern black walnut, walnut

Vital Parts:
Green and black hulls, leaves, twigs

Medicinal Uses:
Taken internally, the green hulls, leaves, and twigs of black walnut have many benefits for the gastrointestinal system. They're great for dispelling parasites, including *giardia* and many worms. Black walnut can also soothe inflammatory bowel disease, hemorrhoids, and other bowel conditions as well as provide relief from constipation and resolve diarrhea. If you're suffering from fungal conditions, such as athlete's foot, jock itch, candida, or ringworm, black walnut applied externally is a great option for treatment. It can also be used to soothe chicken pox, shingles, and cold sores.

Safety Considerations:
Do not use black walnut if you have a tree-nut allergy. Topical use may temporarily stain the skin but is not unsafe.

Preparations:
Standardized extract, tinctures

TIP: Use black walnut as a hair dye for a dark brown color. It dyes fabric well, too! Be sure to wear gloves when you are using this herb, as it will stain your hands.

Blue Vervain

Latin Name: *Verbena hastata*
Common Name(s): Holy herb, simpler's joy, verbena, vervaine

Vital Parts:
Aerial parts in flower

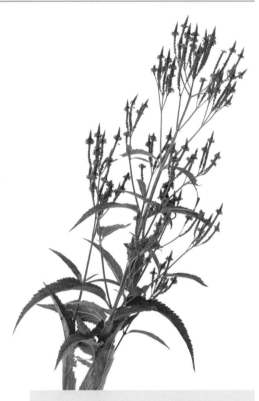

Medicinal Uses:
Blue vervain has been used medicinally in various parts of the world for thousands of years and is known to be one of those herbs that can step in and help at just about any time—meaning it is extremely versatile.

Blue vervain is specific for neck and shoulder pain, with or without tension headache. Another way this ally can provide assistance is by helping you get to sleep when sore and painful muscles make it tough to drift off. The same is true when coughing won't let you sleep.

Safety Considerations:
Large doses can result in upset stomach and vomiting. Avoid if kidney disease is present.

Preparations:
Capsules, teas, tinctures

TIP: As a tincture, the recommended dosage is 25 drops 2 or 3 times a day. For capsules or pills, simply follow the label instructions. As a tea, blue vervain is very bitter, so it's difficult to drink too much, but 3 cups a day is a good guideline.

Boswellia

Latin Name: *Boswellia serrata*
Common Name(s): Indian frankincense

Vital Parts:
Resin

Medicinal Uses:
Boswellia has been used for centuries as an anti-inflammatory and can be used to treat arthritis, rheumatism, and muscle aches. It also helps with other inflammatory diseases like Crohn's disease and ulcerative colitis.

Safety Considerations:
Heartburn, skin rashes, nausea, and diarrhea are occasionally reported by people who take or use boswellia. If purchasing boswellia essential oil, which is typically marketed as frankincense essential oil, be sure that you obtain it from a trusted manufacturer as it is frequently adulterated and sold as perfume oil.

Preparations:
Capsules, creams, essential oil, ointments, salves, tablets

TIP: Boswellia prefers full sun and sandy soil. A native of warm regions in Asia, Africa, and the Middle East, it requires frost-free conditions and cannot survive cold winters. Although boswellia can be grown from seed, you may have better luck with a sapling. Older trees and shrubs do not normally require fertilization, but saplings need supplementation and plenty of water. Once established, boswellia is drought resistant and flourishes in xeriscapes.

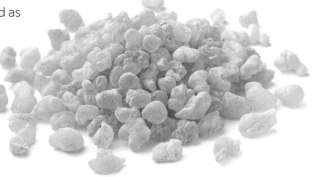

Burdock

Latin Name: *Arctium lappa*
Common Name(s): Beggar's buttons,
burr seed, cocklebur, fox's clote, niu
bang zi, personata, thorny burr

Vital Parts:
Root, seeds, leaves

Medicinal Uses:
Traditionally, burdock is known as an
adaptogen that flushes toxins from the
liver and kidneys. It is a diuretic and can
also be used to promote sweating. In
addition, skin conditions such as psoriasis, eczema, and other itchy rashes, as
well as acne and a dry, irritated scalp,
can all be treated with burdock.

Safety Considerations:
Burdock is generally regarded as
safe. Use caution when separating
seeds because they contain fine hairs
that can irritate the skin—or lungs,
if inhaled.

Preparations:
Compresses, culinary ingredient, decoctions, standardized
extract, tinctures

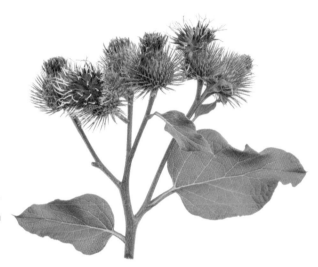

TIP: Dry some leaves to have on hand
during winter. To do this, cut out the
central vein, dry the leaves, then fold,
roll, and store in an airtight jar. Burdock
root is slow and deep working, so it
may take up to 3 months to notice any
healing effects. Because burdock is a
biennial plant, you'll need to harvest
the root between the fall of its first
year and the spring of its second year.

Cacao/Chocolate

Latin Name: *Theobroma cacao*
Common Name(s): Cocoa

Vital Parts:
Unprocessed cocoa, cacao powder, paste, nibs

Medicinal Uses:
Cacao is an ancient superfood that is extremely high in antioxidants, which protect cells from free radicals. It is high in minerals such as magnesium, potassium, iron, chromium, and calcium. Cacao is beneficial to the heart and supports heart health by lowering blood pressure and blood sugar levels. Cacao is also a great mood elevator.

Safety Considerations:
Cacao is generally regarded as safe.

Preparations:
Culinary ingredient, elixirs

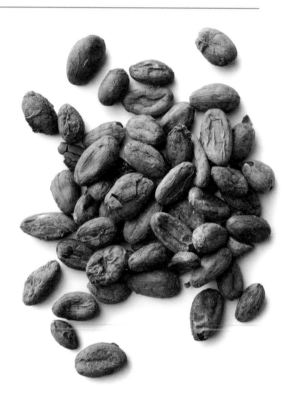

TIP: Unlike cocoa, cacao powder is generally raw and unprocessed with no additives like sugar and dairy. It's made from raw cacao beans that are dried and fermented into cacao nibs, which are then ground into powder.

Calendula

Latin Name: *Calendula officinalis*

Common Name(s): Calendule, common marigold, English garden marigold, Mary bud, Mary's gold, poet's marigold, pot marigold, ruddles, Scotch marigold

Vital Parts:

Flowers and leaves, which contain a sticky resin that is herbal gold, indicating the powerful healing properties held within the plant.

Medicinal Uses:

Calendula is commonly used for skin issues and wounds. It can make a huge difference on foot or leg ulcers, particularly when combined with comfrey. It's also quite useful for digestive and gastrointestinal problems. You can use calendula as a gargle or rinse for the gums and throat. Calendula tea has a history of working as an eyewash to relieve symptoms of pinkeye.

Safety Considerations:

Those allergic to plants in the aster family should avoid calendula. People in early pregnancy should avoid internal use. Otherwise, the herb is considered quite safe for both internal and external use.

Preparations:

Compresses, creams, gels, lotions, poultices, salves, soaps, teas, tinctures

TIP: Calendula is very easy to grow; I simply scatter the seeds in the spring. It's best to cover them with ½ inch of dirt after all danger of frost has passed. They will germinate quickly and bloom from July until frost.

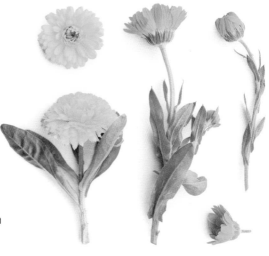

California Poppy

Latin Name: *Eschscholzia californica*
Common Name(s): Cup of gold

Vital Parts:
Aerial parts

Medicinal Uses:
California poppy is a dream come true for those suffering from jerking limbs and restless legs that repeatedly awaken them or disturb their sleep. A dropperful (25 drops) of tincture before bed can help everyone reach a deeper level of sleep. The tea is a nice assist when you're overtired, overwhelmed, cranky, or on the verge of a headache. Externally, the plant can also be applied as a poultice or compress for relief from sciatica pain and throbbing pain. It can also be helpful for PTSD and withdrawal from opiates—however, this usage should always be under the direction of professionals.

Safety Considerations:
Do not combine California poppy with medications for sleep, sedation, or anxiety. Avoid using it during pregnancy or while breastfeeding. Don't drive or operate machinery after ingestion, since this herb can cause drowsiness.

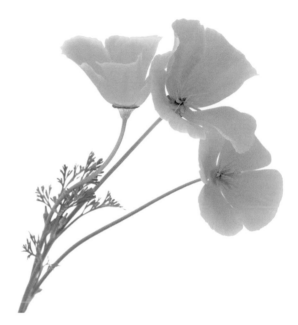

Preparations:
Capsules, compresses, poultices, teas, tinctures

TIP: The recommended dosage is 20 to 30 drops of tincture before bed. Repeat after 30 minutes if needed; tea can also be drunk as needed. It can be bitter, especially with a long brew, so most people won't overdo it.

Capsicum

Latin Name: *Capsicum annuum, Capsicum baccatum, Capsicum chinense, Capsicum frutescens, Capsicum pubescens*

Common Name(s): Cayenne, chile, hot pepper, red pepper

Vital Parts:
Fruit, whole pepper

Medicinal Uses:
Capsicum aids digestion and helps many problems, including upset stomach, intestinal gas, stomach pain, diarrhea, and cramps. The active ingredient, an irritant alkaloid called capsaicin, encourages circulation and thins blood. Some evidence suggests it may help with diabetes and weight management, as well as headaches, blood pressure regulation, and heart disease. Externally, a salve, gel, lotion, or patch on the skin can bring relief to lingering pain post-shingles, the joint pains of osteoarthritis, rheumatoid arthritis, and fibromyalgia, as well as everyday muscle and joint aches.

Safety Considerations:
Avoid external use on children under 2 years of age. Do not apply to broken skin or use near the eyes or mucus membranes. Internal overdose can cause nausea, vomiting, abdominal pain, and burning diarrhea.

Preparations:
Capsules, culinary ingredient, gels, lotions, patches, salves, tinctures

TIP: Peppers are easy to grow from seed. The plants are also becoming popular at nurseries and heirloom herb festivals. Be sure to keep sweet and hot peppers as far apart as possible because they will cross-pollinate, and the heat always wins. Peppers appear on the plant green, turn yellow, then turn orange, ripening to red. Some are purple or brown.

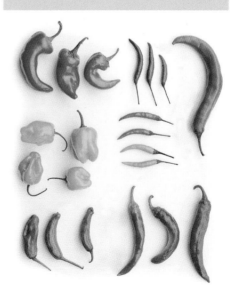

Cardamom

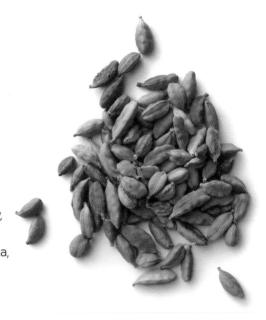

Latin Name: *Elettaria cardamomum*
Common Name(s): Capalaga, Ceylon cardamom, green cardamom, ilachi, true cardamom

Vital Parts:
Whole seeds, ground seeds

Medicinal Uses:
Cardamom is especially good for treating stomach trouble. Traditionally, it has been used to treat a wide range of digestive problems including nausea, diarrhea, poor digestion of fats, gas, bloating, intestinal spasms, stomach cramps, diarrhea, and constipation. It also works preventively to inhibit the growth of bacteria, yeast, and fungi in the gut. Chewing on a whole seed or two after a meal can freshen your breath.

Safety Considerations:
Cardamom is generally regarded as safe.

Preparations:
Capsules, culinary ingredient, essential oil, powdered, teas

TIP: Cardamom is a carminative, meaning it is particularly good at relieving gas buildup in the digestive tract by reducing gas bubbles produced by gut bacteria during digestion. Carminatives also help eliminate intestinal spasms, burping, bloating, and flatulence.

Catnip

Latin Name: *Nepeta cataria*
Common Name(s): Catmint, cat nep, catswort, field balm, herb catta, nep

Vital Parts:

Leaves and flowers before bloom for teas, tincture, vinegar, or any kind of internal application; best while in bloom if insect-repellent properties are desired

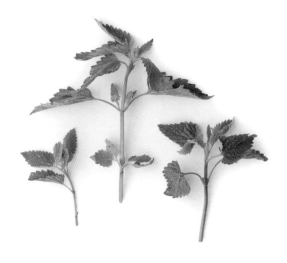

Medicinal Uses:

A cup of tea or a dose of tincture can settle many of the digestive problems brought on by emotional issues, such as cramping and excess gas, and can also help soothe coughing spasms associated with many respiratory issues. Catnip is mild enough to help an overexcited child relax. The essential oil of catnip is a very good mosquito repellent. Essential oil is present in the leaves and flowers of the plants, so rub the undersides (especially) of the leaves and the flowers on skin to shoo away skeeters.

Safety Considerations:

Very large doses may cause vomiting. Avoid catnip while pregnant or if you have kidney or liver issues.

Preparations:

Capsules, essential oils, salves, teas, tinctures

TIP: It's worthwhile to gather some wild blooming catnip during the summer. It takes quite a bit of the fresh herb to dry down to a few ounces.

Chai Blend

Latin Name: *N/A*
Common Name(s): Cha, chai, masala chai
Typical Ingredients: Black tea, milk, sugar, and a wide variety of aromatic herbs and spices such as star anise, black pepper, ginger, cloves, cardamom, cinnamon, and vanilla

Medicinal Uses:

In addition to all the benefits of *Camellia sinensis*, all of the other benefits from the warming spices come into play. You can read about some of them separately among the herbs profiled here. In recent years, herbalists have taken this delicious beverage and created many variations. Sometimes chai doesn't include *Camellia sinensis* at all, and might have rooibos or yerba maté instead. Chai may be made focusing on medicinal mushrooms, specific herbs, or made for a specific medicinal purpose (see Dandelion Chai Mix, page 173). Chai is made by combining about 1 part tea and 1 part hot milk with lots of sweetener.

Safety Considerations:

Tea contains caffeine, so those sensitive to caffeine should avoid it.

Preparations:

Liquid concentrate, teas

TIP: The word *chai* means tea. People often talk about chai tea, which is like saying "tea tea." Most of the time, chai refers to masala chai, with the warming, delicious spices. Generally, only herbalists use the term for other kinds of herbal chai.

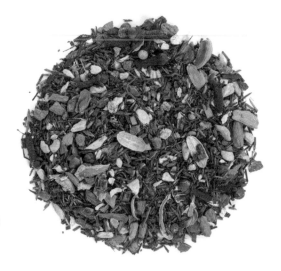

Chamomile

Latin Name: *Matricaria recutita*
(German chamomile)
Common Name(s): Chamomile, earth apple, mantazilla, mayweed

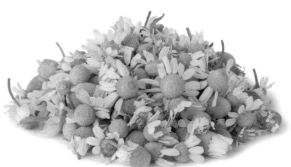

Vital Parts:
Flowers

Medicinal Uses:
I have used very warm tea bags to soothe eye sties, which are staph infections of the eyelids. Having caught them early, I've been a little shocked that they did not progress and by the next day were gone. Chamomile is a delightful remedy for indigestion and cramps because it reduces gas. It calms and relaxes while soothing inflammation in the lower digestive tract and bowel, making it useful for IBS. Try a cup of tea after a meal.

Safety Considerations:
People who have allergies to plants in the aster family may have a problem with chamomile.

Preparations:
Sachets, teas, tinctures

TIP: Chamomile prefers well-drained soil and full sun to part shade with a moderate amount of water—so be sure to water every 3 to 5 days. Weed thoroughly when the plants are getting established, then weed as needed. Fertilize with compost once they are 6 to 8 inches tall. Harvest flowers daily once the plant starts blooming, picking freshly opened blooms in the morning after the dew dries.

Cinnamon

Latin Name: *Cinnamomum verum*
Common Name(s): Canela, cannelle, dalchini, laurus cinnamomum

Vital Parts:
Inner bark, leaves

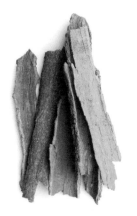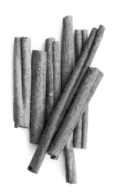

Medicinal Uses:
Cinnamon helps stop vomiting, relieves flatulence, and is useful for getting rid of diarrhea. Some medical doctors are now encouraging their patients to consume cinnamon each day to reduce blood sugar, blood pressure, and cholesterol levels. You can use cinnamon tea for nausea or apply it externally for fungus. Cinnamon essential oil is a potent antibacterial and antifungal ointment.

Preparations:
Capsules, culinary ingredient, essential oils, powdered, teas

TIP: The flavor of freshly grated cinnamon is so much better than the stuff that comes in the jars. I like to grate it at home. It takes a bit of work, but it's worth it. Add it to homemade applesauce—yum!

Safety Considerations:
The coumarin in the cassia variety of cinnamon is a blood thinner, so it is not recommended for individuals on blood-thinner medication. When used in large quantities, such as the daily dosage for medicinal purposes, coumarin is a liver and kidney toxin. Cinnamon essential oil is a skin irritant and somewhat caustic. Always dilute cinnamon essential oil, and opt for leaf oil rather than bark oil.

Clove

Latin Name: *Syzygium aromaticum*
Common Name(s): Clove flower, clove leaf, clove oil, ding xiang, eugenia aromatica, oil of clove

Vital Parts:
Dried flower buds, leaves, and stems

Medicinal Uses:
Clove boosts immunity and treats cold symptoms, including headache, sore throat, fatigue, earache, cough, and congestion. Clove's well-known antiseptic and antimicrobial qualities make it great for use on cuts, wounds, burns, bites, and stings. Clove tea can increase the libido, improve brain function, combat stress, alleviate depression, fight anxiety, reduce memory loss, and treat insomnia. Clove also works wonders on the skin, treating acne, minimizing wrinkles, tightening sagging skin, and combating dryness.

Safety Considerations:
Clove is considered safe when taken in amounts typically found in foods. However, no studies have been done regarding taking the herb for medicinal use in the long term, so children, pregnant people, and those breastfeeding should avoid medicinal doses.

The active ingredient in clove, eugenol, slows blood clotting, so avoid ingesting clove post-surgery or if you're taking blood thinners.

Preparations:
Creams, culinary ingredient, essential oils, ointments, poultices, soaps, teas

TIP: Cloves are the flowering buds of clove trees. They grow easily in wet, tropical areas or rich, red soil. Their ideal conditions are partial shade and rainfall. It takes 20 years for this plant to grow clove buds.

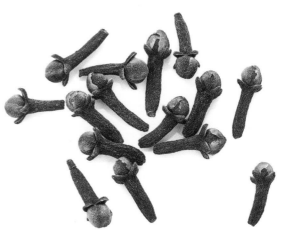

Comfrey

Latin Name: *Symphytum officinale*
Common Name(s): Ass ear, black root, blackwort, gum plant, healing herb, knitback, slippery root, wallwort

Vital Parts:
Root, leaves

Medicinal Uses:
When applied externally, comfrey root helps reduce or eliminate scars and fade age spots. The leaves can be used externally to soothe dry, itchy skin and help heal cuts, perineal tears from childbirth, broken bones, external ulcers, and wounds (when applied in combination with an antimicrobial herb to avoid infection being sealed into the wound). Drink a cup of comfrey leaf tea to soothe and heal gastric and duodenal ulcers, ulcerative colitis, and leaky gut.

Safety Considerations:
Comfrey root should never be taken internally. Do not use comfrey if you have a history of liver conditions or regularly consume alcohol. Comfrey leaves should only be used internally for short periods of time (2 to 4 weeks only). Do not use internally during pregnancy or lactation.

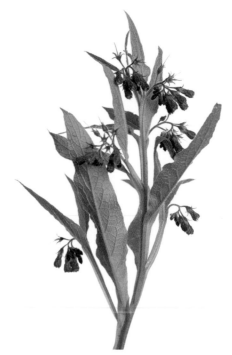

Preparations:
Compresses, poultices, teas

TIP: You'll love comfrey in your garden because its vivid blue and purple flowers look fantastic, it's easy to grow, and it thrives under the shade of other trees and plants. The only downside is that if you ever want to get rid of it, good luck. Its roots are brittle, breakable, and sprout new plants easily.

Dandelion

Latin Name: *Taraxacum officinale*
Common Name(s): Dent de lion,
lion's tooth

Vital Parts:
All parts of the plant except the seeds

Medicinal Uses:
Dandelion helps a wide array of skin
issues, such as acne, dullness, eczema,
bruising, and rashes, by supporting
the liver. It also supports healthy
functioning of the kidneys, spleen,
and gallbladder, and is thought to be
a consistently reliable detoxifying
herb. It is often used to stimulate the
appetite, support digestion, and relieve
excess gas or constipation. The bitter
properties increase bile production, in
turn helping balance blood sugar levels.
Dandelion's diuretic properties make
it an excellent choice for the entire urinary system, including the kidneys and
bladder, cleansing and tonifying without being too drying. Dandelion is also
helpful for symptoms of PMS, relieving pain, and cooling irritability. The
diuretic, pain-relieving, and detoxifying
abilities also help with gout and edema.

Safety Considerations:
Dandelion is generally regarded as safe.

Preparations:
Capsules, culinary ingredient, salves,
teas, tinctures, vinegars

TIP: You may like the bitter flavor of
dandelion, but you can shade the plant
in order to blanch it, which produces a
milder flavor. A relative kept a wooden
frame around a patch of dandelions,
with boards on top to shield it from the
sun. The plants stayed pale and mild
into early summer.

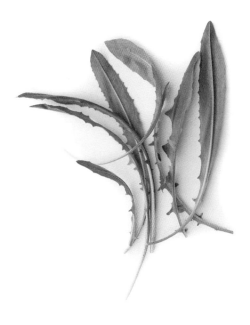

Echinacea

Latin Name: *E. angustifolia* and
E. purpurea most often
Common Name(s): Black Sampson,
Indian head, purple coneflower, red
sunflower, snakeroot

Vital Parts:
All parts of the plant are
medicinal—from root to flower

Medicinal Uses:
Echinacea can help heal toothaches,
snakebites, stings, allergies, wounds,
burns, joint pain, sore throats, coughs,
colds, and infections. It boosts the
immune system and attacks general
infection; treats weeping wounds, boils,
abscesses, urinary tract infections, and
enlarged lymph glands; promotes skin
regeneration; and ameliorates psoriasis. You can take it both internally and
externally for many of these afflictions,
thereby multiplying the effects.

Safety Considerations:
Some people are allergic to echinacea,
so use caution if you have other known
plant allergies. Large, frequent doses
can cause nausea. Some people don't
need to take large doses for this side
effect to occur. Avoid in the case of
autoimmune disease.

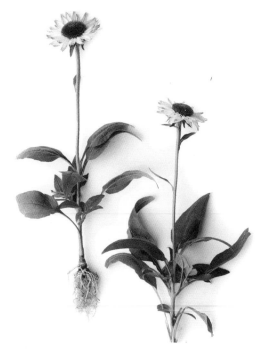

Preparations:
Capsules, compresses, cough drops,
poultices, salves, syrups, teas, tinctures

TIP: Every year I pull a plant and clean
the roots carefully before grinding
them, along with some leaves and a
flower or two, to mix with high-proof
vodka in a jar. A good tincture made
with fresh roots will have a little tingle
on the tongue.

Elder

Latin Name: *Sambucus canadensis, Sambucus cerulean, Sambucus nigra*
Common Name(s): Black elder, elderberry, European black elderberry, European elder, European elderberry, Mexican elderberry. Blossoms are sometimes referred to as "elder blow."

Vital Parts:
Fresh cooked (not raw) or dried berries, flowers

Medicinal Uses:
Elderberries are antiviral, diaphoretic, diuretic, and laxative. They are also a good source of anthocyanins, which are powerful antioxidants. They contain vitamins A and C, calcium, thiamine, niacin, potassium, and protein. Elderberries can help prevent colds and flu and relieve congestion. Like elderberries, elderflower is also anti-inflammatory, antiviral, and assists the body in removing excess mucus. One of elderflower's best-known abilities is in bringing on a sweat. It is very often used for beauty treatments or to help with myriad skin issues, from rosacea to diaper rash.

Safety Considerations:
Elderberries and elderflower are generally regarded as safe.

Preparations:
Cough drops, culinary ingredient, flower essences, syrups, teas, tinctures, wines

TIP: When the berries ripen, it can be overwhelming to harvest them all. Some go directly into the freezer in the right quantity for syrup, while the bulk is made into juice by heating the berries with a little lemon juice. Use a fork to easily remove the berries from the stem when harvesting them.

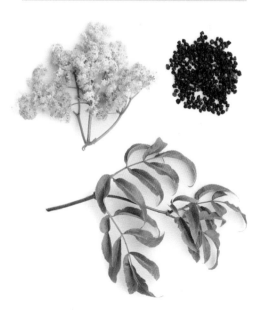

Eleuthero

Latin Name:
Eleutherococcus senticosus
Common Name(s): Eleuthero,
Siberian ginseng

Vital Parts:
Root mostly; less often, leaves

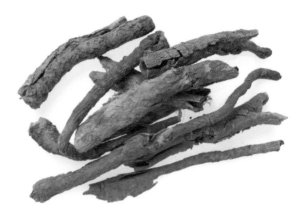

Medicinal Uses:
Eleuthero was the first adaptogen I ever worked with. At the time it generally went by the name Siberian ginseng, and it has been an amazing ally for me. Eleuthero is ideal for addressing anxiety, sluggish brain function, a cold, fatigue, the flu, herpes, and stress. For fatigue and a dread of the daily grind, try taking eleuthero for a month. Stop for a week and then take for another month. Evaluate from there. Eleuthero can be helpful for tackling big or super-boring tasks, providing stamina and the ability to stay focused.

Preparations:
Capsules, powder, tablets, teas, tinctures

TIP: The recommended dosage as a tincture is 30 to 50 drops 1 to 3 times a day. Follow label instructions for capsules.

Safety Considerations:
Although side effects are rare, eleuthero should be avoided in high doses by individuals with very high blood pressure, insomnia, irritability, melancholy, and anxiety.

Eucalyptus

Latin Name: *Eucalyptus globulus*
Common Name(s): Blue gum, fever tree, gully gum, red gum, stringy bark tree

Vital Parts:
Leaves and oil

Medicinal Uses:
Eucalyptus has been used traditionally to treat fever, coughs, and congestion as well as to ameliorate respiratory problems and asthma. It is well known for its ability to alleviate osteoarthritis pain and joint pain. It can also be used for upset stomach, liver and gallbladder issues, ulcers, burns, wounds, depression, and to fight acne.

Safety Considerations:
Eucalyptus should be diluted before applying topically to skin. If you suffer from diabetes, note that eucalyptus has been shown in studies to lower blood sugar. Do not ingest eucalyptus essential oil; ingest products made only with whole leaves. Eucalyptus interacts with several pharmaceuticals. If taking prescription medication, check to ensure no adverse reaction is indicated.

Preparations:
Capsules, compresses, essential oils, gels, ointments, salves, splashes

TIP: Growing eucalyptus indoors is easy and quite common. It needs full sunlight and well-drained soil. Keep temps between 50°F and 75°F. If you're planting outdoors, heads-up that this tree won't reach its full height potential unless you live in a warm climate.

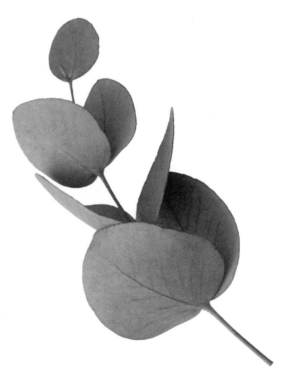

Fennel

Latin Name: *Foeniculum vulgare,*
F. vulgare azoricum
Common Name(s): Bitter fennel,
common fennel, Florence fennel,
Roman fennel, sweet anise,
sweet fennel

Vital Parts:
Seed, bulb, leaf, stalk

Medicinal Uses:
When a breastfeeding person drinks
a cup of fennel tea, it can stimulate
breast milk production and prevent
mastitis. When it passes to baby, it
helps reduce teething pain. Diluted
fennel tea given to baby treats colic
as well. Fennel works against gas,
bloating, flatulence, nausea, and
vomiting and treats intestinal viruses.
It can also alleviate a dry cough and
loosen congestion.

Safety Considerations:
Fennel is generally regarded as safe,
though large doses can overstimulate
the nervous system. Avoid during pregnancy in more than culinary amounts.

Preparations:
Culinary ingredient, teas, tinctures

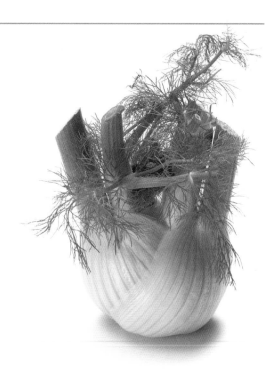

TIP: Fennel is a perennial that grows
to a height of 8 feet. The plant prefers
full sun to part shade in well-drained
soil and is drought tolerant once
established. Fennel does not like trans-
planting. So, if growing from seed, sow
directly or plant in a compostable pot
that can be directly planted. Trim off
dead growth at the end of the growing
season. Harvest seeds once they turn
brown on the stalk. Harvest leaves and
stalks during the growing season. Harvest bulbs in late summer or fall.

Feverfew

Latin Name: *Tanacetum parthenium*
Common Name(s): Bachelor's buttons, featherfew

Vital Parts:
Leaves, buds, and flowers

Medicinal Uses:
Feverfew is traditionally used for the treatment of fevers, rheumatoid arthritis, stomachaches, toothaches, insect bites, infertility, and problems with menstruation and labor during childbirth. Feverfew can also be taken to prevent migraines or to alleviate nausea brought on by a migraine.

Safety Considerations:
Pregnant people should not take feverfew. Those who take therapeutic doses of aspirin or prescription blood thinners should avoid it as well, as it can increase the risk of bleeding. If you take feverfew on a regular basis to prevent migraines and stop abruptly, you may experience withdrawal headaches. If stopping feverfew, taper off slowly to avoid this uncomfortable side effect.

Preparations:
Capsules, standardized extract, teas

TIP: Among the easiest herbs to grow, feverfew may be propagated by planting seeds directly into disturbed soil or dividing roots from established plants. It requires well-drained soil but does not normally need fertilizer of any kind. Though it prefers full sun, it will tolerate light shade. If you rely on fresh feverfew for migraine prevention, keep a few potted feverfew plants indoors during the winter months.

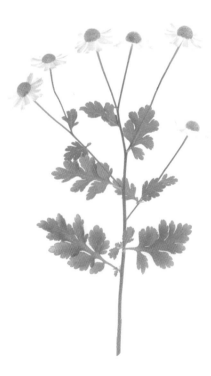

Garlic

Latin Name: *Allium sativum*
Common Name(s): Stinking rose

Vital Parts:
Bulbs, cloves, scapes, flowers

Medicinal Uses:
Garlic clears arteries, thins blood, heals wounds, treats lung ailments, and combats bacteria and yeast. It helps fight coughs, heart ailments, high blood pressure, and high cholesterol and regulates blood sugar. Eating garlic can also prevent flea, tick, and mosquito bites.

Safety Considerations:
If you're on blood-thinning medication, check with your doctor before taking garlic medicinally. Also, let your physician know about garlic supplementation before surgery so they can tell you when to stop taking it. Garlic supplementation (above dietary use) should be avoided during pregnancy. Garlic may cause contact dermatitis with overuse.

Preparations:
Capsules, culinary ingredient, infused oils, juices, pills, poultices, tinctures

TIP: Garlic is easy to grow and doesn't take much space. If you have a source of garlic, purchase a bulb to grow. Plant in autumn or early spring, in a sunny location with well-drained soil. Plant root-side down 4 to 6 inches apart in rows 1 to 2 inches apart. Cover with 2 inches of dirt. Mulch for winter.

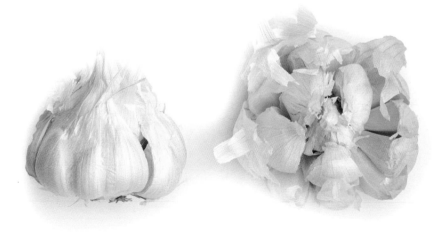

Geranium

Latin Name: *Pelargonium*
Common Name(s): Cranesbill, spotted cranesbill, wild geranium, wood geranium

Vital Parts:
Roots

Medicinal Uses:
Geranium is used to treat digestive conditions, IBS, and hemorrhoids. It also balances hormones and regulates menstruation and vaginal discharge. Geranium can improve moods and detoxify the body. It also is useful for treating canker sores and gum disease. A powerful astringent, geranium is known for opening, cleaning, and shrinking the size of your pores.

Safety Considerations:
Geranium is usually well tolerated and is generally considered safe, but some people are sensitive to it, reporting mild gastrointestinal upset, rashes, itching, and swelling. Safety has not been established for use by pregnant or nursing people.

Preparations:
Creams, oils, shampoos, splashes, teas, tinctures, toners, tonics

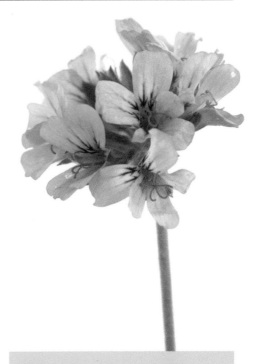

TIP: Geraniums are fairly easy to grow and able to withstand a variety of harsh conditions like drought or heat. Their perfect situation is full sunlight, warm temps, and a covered location, making it ideal for a windowsill indoors. You can grow them from seed or cuttings.

Ginger

Latin Name: *Zingiber officinale*
Common Name(s): Awapuhi, ginger root

Vital Parts:
Root

Medicinal Uses:
Ginger is best known for its ability to help nausea, including sea sickness, chemotherapy-related nausea, nausea after surgery, and morning sickness in pregnancy. It also stimulates digestion, causing the stomach to empty faster while soothing and relaxing the entire system. Ginger may also help with menstrual pain, migraine headaches, and gum health. Regular use of ginger may help relieve pain and swelling from osteoarthritis, rheumatoid arthritis, and muscular pains.

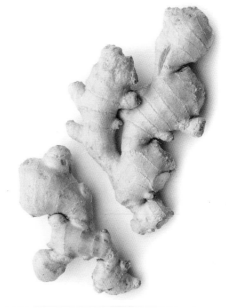

Safety Considerations:
Ginger thins the blood, so if you are on anticoagulant medicines, use it in moderation. More than 1 teaspoon of powder or 1 tablespoon fresh may cause heartburn.

Preparations:
Baths, crystallized, culinary ingredient, fresh, pickled, powdered, syrups, teas, tinctures

TIP: You can grow ginger indoors as long as you have a very warm spot, like a window with clear southern exposure. Give each plant a 12- to 18-inch pot with good drainage. Place trimmed rhizomes eye- or bud-up, and cover with an inch or so of good dirt.

Ginkgo

Latin Name: *Ginkgo biloba*
Common Name(s): Maidenhair

Vital Parts:
Leaves mostly; nuts in some parts of the world

Medicinal Uses:
Ginkgo is ideal for addressing circulation problems, memory loss, Alzheimer's disease symptoms, glaucoma, vertigo, tinnitus, hearing loss, and sexual dysfunction. It is believed to improve blood flow throughout the brain, including the small capillaries, so that the brain is healthier and oxygenated.

Safety Considerations:
Though generally recognized as safe, ginkgo may cause bleeding when taken in conjunction with blood-thinning medications and medications for high blood pressure and diabetes. Check with your doctor before taking ginkgo. Pregnant people should not take ginkgo in any form.

Preparations:
Capsules, pills, standardized extract, tinctures

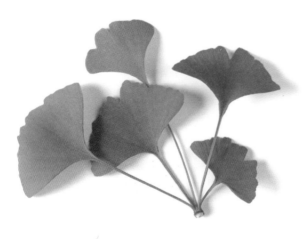

TIP: Ginkgo trees are hardy and capable of thriving in most backyards throughout North America and the rest of the world. Leaves are harvested after they reach maturity but before they begin to change color as days begin to grow shorter. Use caution if you decide to grow a ginkgo tree or two, as the nuts are protected by a fleshy, orange fruit-like coating that causes contact dermatitis similar to the stinging rash caused by poison ivy. The nuts come only from the female tree, and are notorious for their awful smell. However, it can take 20 years before you can tell which sex tree you have.

Ginseng

Latin Name: *Panax ginseng*
Common Name(s): American ginseng, Canadian ginseng, panax quinquefolia, red berry, ren shen, shang, shi yang seng

Vital Parts:
Roots

Medicinal Uses:
Ginseng is a major force in strengthening immunity and treating digestive, heart, and nervous system issues. It's a powerful addition to an antiaging beauty regimen, as it stimulates cell turnover and hair growth, evens skin tone, smooths texture, and treats under-eye wrinkles and dark circles. Specifically, ginseng treats flu, colds, diabetes, depression, anxiety, anemia, nerve pain, and fatigue. It also stops the hardening of arteries; triggers metabolism; stabilizes blood sugar, mood, mental health, and insulin levels; and lowers cholesterol.

Safety Considerations:
Because ginseng can cause blood sugar to drop, it is not recommended for people with diabetes. Those with hypertension should also avoid the herb, as it can cause blood pressure to increase significantly. Overuse can lead to anxiety, insomnia, and digestive discomfort.

Preparations:
Capsules, standardized extract, tea

TIP: Got 5 to 10 years? That's how long it takes ginseng to reach maturity before you harvest it. Your best bet is to buy older roots—say 3 to 4 years old—and plant them in spring. They prefer shade beneath other tree canopies and moist, well-drained soils.

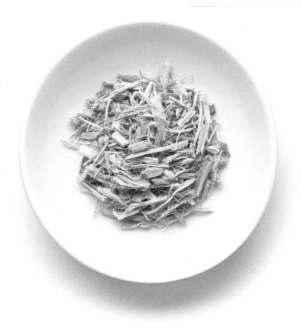

Goldenseal

Latin Name: *Hydrastis canadensis*
Common Name(s): Chinese golden-seal, eye balm, eye root, goldenroot, hydraste, Indian plant, Indian turmeric

Vital Parts:
Roots or rhizomes

Medicinal Uses:
The main active ingredients in goldenseal—berberine and beta-hydrastine—have massive antimicrobial and astringent benefits, not to mention it's a powerful anti-bacterial, antiviral, and decongestant. Goldenseal treats acne, skin infections and irritation, bronchitis, digestive problems, colds, flus, reproductive issues, eye infections, mouth issues, eczema, psoriasis, external wounds, and ulcers. It also helps protect the liver, fights cancer, lowers cholesterol, and boosts immunity.

Safety Considerations:
Goldenseal should not be taken internally for longer than three weeks consecutively. It is not appropriate for use by those suffering from hypogly-cemia or high blood pressure. Because goldenseal can cause uterine contrac-tions, it should not be used by people

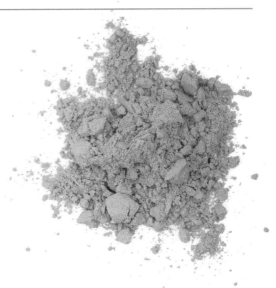

who are pregnant or lactating, or by infants. Do not take it in conjunction with prescription medication.

Preparations:
Capsules, ointments, salves, standard-ized extract, teas

TIP: Because goldenseal is a native of forested areas in Canada and the eastern United States, it thrives in similar climates and conditions: three-quarters shade and beneath a large tree. Soil should be humus rich. That said, even if you get its garden-ing demands correct, you still have a 3-year wait for a harvest.

Gotu Kola

Latin Name: *Centella asiatica*
Common Name(s): Asiatic pennywort, Indian pennywort

Vital Parts:
Aerial parts

Medicinal Uses:
Externally, gotu kola is applied to reduce age spots, stimulate collagen production, and heal scars, wounds, burns, bed sores, and ulcers. It also can encourage skin graft healing. Internally, gotu kola is a great brain tonic, helping restore and improve memory and concentration, and calming the mind. As a nervous system supportive, gotu kola helps with nervous breakdown, neuralgia, and depression. Gotu kola also has been used to treat varicose veins, jaundice, and macular degeneration and other visual weaknesses. It can aid with fatigue and a wide range of diseases, including malaria, tuberculosis, syphilis, leprosy, lupus, sexually transmitted diseases (STD), and encephalitis.

Safety Considerations:
Generally regarded as safe, though large doses may cause dizziness, headache, itching, stupor, and vertigo. Can also be stimulating to the thyroid, so avoid in cases of hyperthyroidism.

Preparations:
Oil infusions, teas, tinctures

TIP: Gotu kola is easy to grow if it has plenty of water. Plant it in a mini water garden and keep it moist.

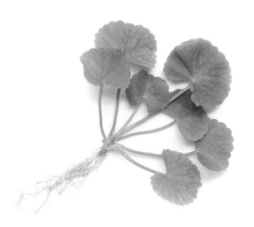

Hawthorn

Latin Name: *Crataegus laevigata*
Common Name(s): Cockspur, cockspur thorn, English hawthorn, haw, maybush, may tree, quickset, red haw, summer haw, thornapple, Washington thorn, whitethorn

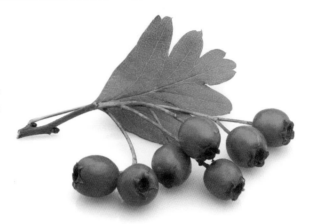

Vital Parts:
Berries, leaves, and flowers

Medicinal Uses:
Hawthorn is terrific for all things heart-related. It helps the body heal from heart attacks, heart muscle weakness, degenerative heart disease, irregular heartbeats, and congestive heart failure; stabilizes angina; and speeds recuperation from heart surgery. Hawthorn helps open up circulation, reduces effects of hardening of the arteries, lowers blood pressure, and protects the body from free radicals that contribute to heart disease. It also calms the nervous system, helping in times of grief and heartbreak. Hawthorn improves concentration and focus for children with ADD. It strengthens and protects joint lining, collagen, and spinal disks and assists in the digestion of greasy food, fats, and meats.

Safety Considerations:
If taking heart medications, check with your doctor before using hawthorn because it can interfere with or increase their effectiveness.

Preparations:
Capsules, pills, teas, tinctures

TIP: The recommended dosage depends on the ailment. For prevention tincture: 20 to 30 drops 3 times a day. For capsules and pills, follow directions on the label.

Hibiscus

Latin Name: *Hibiscus sabdariffa*
Common Name(s): Roselle, rose mallow

Vital Parts:
Calyx (fruit) and flowers

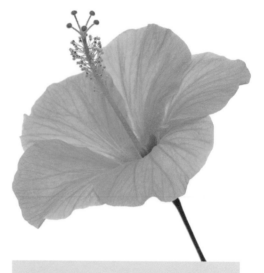

Medicinal Uses:
Hibiscus is loaded with vitamin C. Hibiscus flowers are a great source of antioxidants, which play a role in promoting heart health and lowering blood pressure. It also has some diuretic qualities and is cooling and anti-inflammatory.

Safety Considerations:
Hibiscus has no known side effects; however, people taking diuretics should use it sparingly. If you suffer from heart disease or high blood pressure, check with your health-care provider before using hibiscus. It should not be used by people who are pregnant or lactating.

Preparations:
Capsules, teas, tinctures

TIP: Hibiscus is cultivated in warm and tropical climates where frost is nonexistent or rare. Hibiscus calyxes are typically marketed as hibiscus fruit and can be found in health-food stores as well as at online retailers. Teas, tinctures, and other formulated herbal medicines containing hibiscus are readily available from a variety of sources, including many major retailers.

Holy Basil

Latin Name: *Ocimum tenuiflorum*
Common Name(s): Hot basil, incomparable one, Indian basil, ocimum sanctum, queen of herbs, sacred basil, tulasi, tulsi

Vital Parts:
Aerial parts

Medicinal Uses:
Holy basil supports the immune system. It also helps combat cold and flu symptoms by reducing fever and treating bronchitis, earache, and headache. Holy basil can be used to help alleviate emotional distress including anxiety, depression, and stress. It can also be used to repel mosquitos and for skin issues such as eczema, hives, and ringworm.

Safety Considerations:
If you're taking an anticoagulant, check with your physician before using holy basil. Stop use of the herb before surgery. Hypoglycemic people may experience drops in blood sugar and should use holy basil with caution.

Preparations:
Capsules, culinary ingredient, essential oils, teas, tinctures

TIP: In my region, zone 6b, holy basil grows as an annual. In tropical climates, it will grow like shrubs with woody stems. I usually plant a short row of holy basil plants, but be warned—birds love them. I cover mine with netting until they are about 8 to 10 inches tall; otherwise, the birds will get to them before I do!

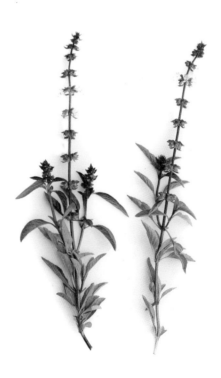

Hops

Latin Name: *Humulus lupulus*
Common Name(s): Common hop

Vital Parts:
Strobiles

Medicinal Uses:
Over the years, hops has been shown to be effective at triggering weight loss, treating menstrual symptoms, soothing anxiety, and balancing moods. It's used today to treat and moisturize over-worked, dry, or irritated skin. Hops treats anxiety; insomnia; ADHD; mood issues like irritability, tension, excitability; stom-ach cramps; nerve pain; and indigestion. It also balances hormones, promotes sleep, and detoxes the liver.

Safety Considerations:
Hops is considered safe and nontoxic. However, some people should take care when using it because it can worsen depression. It also simulates estrogen, so avoid hops if you've been diagnosed with breast cancer. Do not take hops before driving, operating machinery, or performing tasks that require your full attention.

Preparations:
Capsules, culinary ingredient, teas, tinctures

TIP: Hops plants are fairly easy to grow, and since they are sturdy climb-ers, they can be grown against a fence or on a trellis. The hops plant requires rich, well-drained soil and plenty of sunlight to thrive. Obtain rhizomes from a garden store, brewer's supply store, or other reliable source, plant them 1 foot deep and 3 feet apart against a fence or other support in early spring and keep them watered.

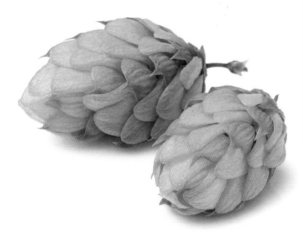

Horse Chestnut

Latin Name: *Aesculus hippocastanum*
Common Name(s): Buckeye, conker tree, European horse chestnut

Vital Parts:
Flowers, seeds, leaves, and bark

Medicinal Uses:
Horse chestnut has been used externally to treat leg and joint pain, varicose veins, itching or swelling in the legs and leg cramps, fever, bladder and gastrointestinal problems, and fluid retention.

Safety Considerations:
Horse chestnuts should only be used externally. Although they are eaten by some animals, they are poisonous to humans. Do not apply horse chestnut products to broken or ulcerated skin. Several high-quality horse chestnut products are available commercially; these have been processed to remove toxins.

Preparations:
Creams, ointments, salves, standardized extract

TIP: Be extremely cautious about growing horse chestnut trees to use in your herbal medicines. They are primarily valued for their stately beauty. These trees require full sun and rich, moist, well-drained soil. You can obtain them from nurseries or plant the seeds yourself; give them a large space in which to grow and they will provide shade and visual interest for years to come.

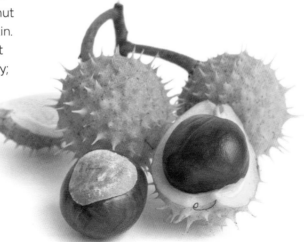

Horseradish

Latin Name: *Armoracia rusticana*
Common Name(s): Stingnose

Vital Parts:
Fresh root, small young leaves, and flowers

Medicinal Uses:
Horseradish stimulates the gallbladder's release of bile, making it a great alternative treatment for digestive problems. All head colds and stuck upper-respiratory infections respond to horseradish. It is also helpful with arthritis, urinary tract infections, headaches, kidney stones, fluid retention, cough, bronchitis, sore muscles, sciatic nerve pain, and gout. Horseradish is thought to detoxify the liver. Syrups help hoarseness or bronchitis specifically but are useful for other applications as well. Young leaves can be used as instant poultices for headaches and laid directly on the forehead. The fresh flowers may be made into a tea as an antiviral and a mild decongestant.

Safety Considerations:
Horseradish essential oil is classified as a hazardous substance, and the juice can cause blistering, so check skin frequently when using the root in a poultice.

Preparations:
Culinary ingredient, poultices, syrups, teas, tinctures, vinegars

> **TIP:** Horseradish is easy to grow, and it will spread. In some cases, it can be downright invasive. Mine is in the shade, and while it has increased from one crown to about six over a decade, that's not terrible. Never rototill horseradish.

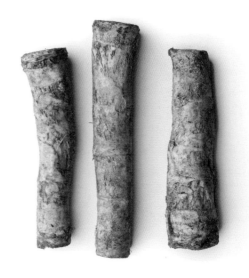

Hyssop

Latin Name: *Hyssopus officinalis*
Common Name(s): Herbe de Joseph, hiope, hysope, jufa, ysop

Vital Parts:
Aerial parts

Medicinal Uses:
Hyssop is used for sore throats, colds and congestion, hoarseness, coughs, and mild asthma. It can be helpful for urinary tract inflammations. It is good for the whole digestive system, assisting in appetite stimulation, colic, and excess gas. It calms nervousness and anxiety, and stops spasms of the lungs and gut. Hyssop has several illness-busting properties, meaning it can fight viral infections and bacterial infections and ease inflammation. It encourages perspiration to help break a fever. It is sometimes used externally on wounds and insect bites. Hyssop is revered in ritual and healing, and is well-known as a purifier physically, emotionally, and spiritually.

Safety Considerations:
Pregnant people should avoid hyssop essential oil. It's packed with ketones, which may cause uterine cramps or trigger the onset of menstruation. Never take hyssop essential oil internally. Hyssop may also spur the onset of or heighten seizures.

Preparations:
Compresses, poultices, syrups, teas, tinctures

> **TIP:** Hyssop blooms from June through October and is generally considered to be evergreen. It is extremely easy to grow and a pretty plant, too.

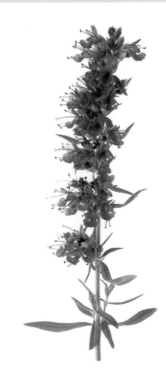

Juniper

Latin Name: *Juniperus communis*
Common Name(s): Common or dwarf juniper

Vital Parts:
Berries

Medicinal Uses:
Juniper's antirheumatic qualities make it great for treating arthritis and rheumatism. It is also an antiseptic commonly used to treat acne, bronchitis, dermatitis, eczema, gout, and psoriasis. Its diuretic qualities make it helpful for treating urinary tract infections and water retention.

Safety Considerations:
Pregnant people should avoid herbal medicines containing juniper, as the plant is a known abortifacient. Those who suffer from kidney disease or kidney infections should not use juniper.

Preparations:
Capsules, culinary ingredient, decoctions, essential oils, tinctures

TIP: The easiest way to grow juniper is to obtain a tree or two from a nursery, as the tree is notoriously difficult to grow from seed. Juniper trees prefer well-drained soil and tend to do best when gravel and rocks are present. The fruiting bodies ripen on a two-year cycle; pick the ones that are dark colored and leave the green ones behind.

Kava

Latin Name: *Piper methysticum, Piper wichmanii*
Common Name(s): Awa, kava-kava

Vital Parts:
Roots

Medicinal Uses:
Kava is an anesthetic, relaxant, and sedative. It's commonly used to treat anxiety, irritability, and menopause symptoms.

Safety Considerations:
Do not take kava with alcohol or use kava products that have been processed with alcohol. In addition, do not take kava if you use acetaminophen or prescription medications, as serious liver damage can result.

Preparations:
Aqueous extract, capsules, teas

TIP: Supplements containing kava are available at some major retailers as well as health-food stores and from reputable online sources. Unless you live in a tropical region or have a greenhouse, you will not be able to grow kava. It must be propagated from rootstock or stem cuttings. Free movement of both moisture and air around the plant is essential. It is easiest to purchase quality kava for making herbal medicine.

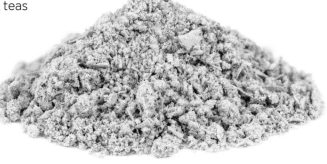

Lady's Mantle

Latin Name: *Alchemilla vulgaris* aka *Alchemilla mollis*
Common Name(s): Dew cup, lion's foot, little alchemist, parsley piert

Vital Parts:
Leaves and flowers

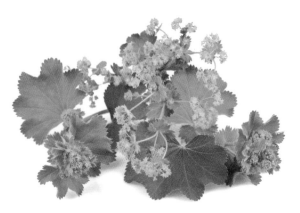

Medicinal Uses:
Lady's mantle is best known for assisting with all kinds of complaints, from PMS by getting rid of excess water and bloating, to cooling and soothing nerves in menopause by aiming to correct hormonal imbalances. There is a high amount of tannin in lady's mantle, making it good when toning, cooling, and drying up excess fluid are called for in a remedy. Otherwise, it is just as helpful for inflammation, diarrhea, and other gastrointestinal complaints, as well as sore throats and spasms. A wash made like a strong tea will speed healing of wounds, rashes, and many skin complaints.

Preparations:
Compresses, teas, tinctures, washes

> **TIP:** Prepare 2 teaspoons of dried herb in a tea or infusion, or 20 to 40 drops tincture that can be taken up to 3 times daily.

Safety Considerations:
Not recommended for use by those who are pregnant or breastfeeding.

Lavender

Latin Name: *Lavandula angustifolia or Lavender* spp.
Common Name(s): Lavandula; common, English, French, garden, spike, sweet, and true lavender

Vital Parts:
Flowers, although all aerial parts are potent

Medicinal Uses:
The heady aromatics of fresh or dried lavender and the herbal constituents combine for a remedy that relaxes muscles and eases spasms that accompany muscular pain. A tea, tincture, or vinegar can help digestion, gas, nausea, and intestinal cramping. The herb in a sachet encourages sleep and helps with tension headaches. Topically, lavender tea, balm, or vinegar can help treat fungal infections, wounds, eczema, and varicose ulcers; soothe sunburned or windburned skin; heal burns; and calm acne. Lavender is a great herb for easing menstrual cramps, tension, and depression, and in menopause can help with insomnia.

Safety Considerations:
There are no known precautions for the herb. However, overuse or undiluted use of the essential oil has been known to sensitize the user, which can be debilitating.

Preparations:
Culinary ingredient, essential oils, infused oils, sachets, teas, tinctures, topical, vinegars

TIP: Depending on your growing zone, different species or cultivars will be hardy, although those in zones 5 or below may not be able to keep lavender outside over the winter.

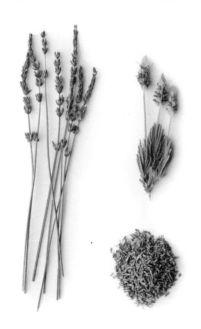

Lemon Balm

Latin Name: *Melissa officinalis*
Common Name(s): Bee balm, English balm, honey plant, lemon balm, Melissa balm, sweet balm

Vital Parts:
Leaves, best before flowering

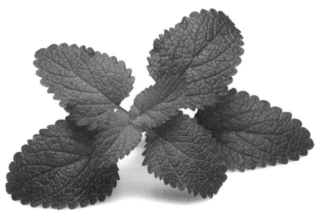

Medicinal Uses:
Lemon balm is commonly used for nervous system complaints, such as nervousness, anxiety, stress, headaches caused by nervous tension, agitation (especially for those with Alzheimer's disease, dementia, and ADHD), stress-related digestive complaints, and illnesses that affect the nervous system, including chronic fatigue and depression. Along with these benefits, it improves concentration and cognitive function, increases flow of bile in the liver, aids in fighting off viruses, and lowers blood pressure. When used externally, lemon balm repels mosquitoes and other insects.

Preparations:
Glycerite, hydrosol, infused oils, powder, salves, teas, tinctures, vinegars

> **TIP:** The key to getting lemon balm growing is to make sure you get a couple of plants started and it will self sow. Ideal for zones 4 to 9, it prefers moist soil and full to partial sun.

Safety Considerations:
Lemon balm is considered safe except for those with hypothyroidism or low thyroid activity. Those on thyroid medication should check with their doctor before using lemon balm.

Licorice

Latin Name: *Glycyrrhiza glabra*
Common Name(s): Drop, gan zao, sweet root

Vital Parts:
Dried root

Medicinal Uses:
Licorice promotes excretion of dry, stuck mucus, and can also ease bronchitis. It soothes the entire gastrointestinal system, including ailments such as heartburn, GERD, ulcers, and constipation and is also considered helpful for adrenal fatigue. It's one of the most commonly used herbs in traditional Chinese medicine, as it is believed to guide other herbs to their best healing expression.

Safety Considerations:
The active ingredient glycyrrhizic acid can stress the kidneys and heart due to its potential to deplete potassium and retain sodium. Avoid licorice in pregnancy. Individuals with high blood pressure, liver disorders, water retention, renal insufficiency, low blood potassium, or heart disease should also avoid this herb.

Preparations:
Capsules, culinary ingredient, pastilles, teas, tinctures

TIP: During cooler weather when germs fly around, I use a licorice root stick in almost every medicinal tea I drink. Simply pop it in the mug and let it stand as the tea steeps. Even if you don't care for black licorice candy, try a cup of tea. It's delicious and so soothing!

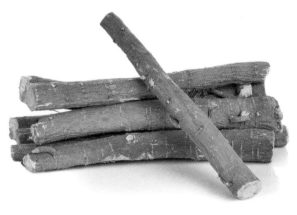

Linden

Latin Name: *Tilia* spp.
Common Name(s): Basswood, lime flower, lime tree, tilia

Vital Parts:
The flowers with the attached leaflike bract

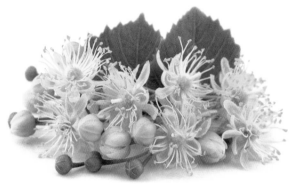

Medicinal Uses:
Restlessness, insomnia, hyperactivity in children, nervous and muscle tension, anxiety, and headaches (especially migraines) all respond well to linden. The mucilage produced by the plant soothes digestive issues and may also help calm irritated membranes in the mouth or throat and decrease mucus production. Linden also relieves muscle spasms and cramps and improves circulation. One of the most noted uses of linden is in inducing perspiration for feverish colds, flu, and infections. It also helps reduce nasal congestion and calm coughs. Externally, you can use linden as a wash or lotion for itchy skin.

Preparations:
Lotions, syrups, teas, tinctures, vinegars

TIP: Harvest linden in early summer, when the fragrant flowers are just beginning to bloom, picking the flowers along with the pale green bract. While in bloom, the tree will most likely be buzzing with bees—they love linden and make a tasty honey from the flowers.

Safety Considerations:
Excessive use has, in rare cases, been associated with heart damage in individuals with heart disease. If you have a heart condition, talk to your doctor before using.

Marshmallow

Latin Name: *Althaea officinalis*
Common Name(s): Cheeses, common marshmallow, mallards, mallow, mortification root, sweet weed, white mallow

Vital Parts:
Mainly root; also flowers and leaves

Medicinal Uses:
Marshmallow is ideal for addressing bronchitis, burns, constipation, dry cough, diarrhea, heartburn, reflux, skin irritation, sore throat, stomach, urinary tract inflammation, ulcerative colitis, and ulcers. The very slippery, soothing mucilage that is created with marshmallow and liquid is perfect for soothing mucus membranes throughout the entire digestive system. Infuse it in cool or room-temperature water overnight, and drink the thick, soothing beverage in the morning. If the texture is an issue, blend it with a few other things—like bananas, yogurt, and so on.

Safety Considerations:
Drink a full glass of water (or tea) when taking marshmallow. It may interfere with some medications, particularly those treating blood sugar. Wait an hour between taking marshmallow and other medications.

Preparations:
Capsules, creams, dried, lotions, poultices, syrups, teas, tinctures

TIP: Wash the roots well. Chop, then dry them on trays or in a dehydrator. Lay leaves or flowers flat to dry. In a pinch, flowers and leaves of okra, hollyhock, and rose of Sharon can be used similarly to marshmallow.

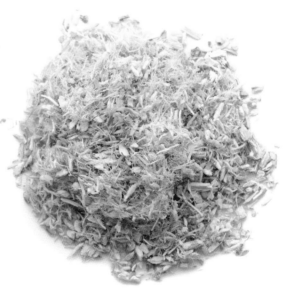

Matcha

Latin Name: *Camellia sinensis*
Common Name(s): Maccha

Vital Parts:
Only the tender new leaves, which are dried and ground to a fine powder

Medicinal Uses:
The antibacterial, anti-inflammatory, and astringent properties of matcha make it an excellent choice for skin issues like acne, rashes, and uneven areas. There is also a light exfoliating, scrubby texture that leaves skin glowing. Green tea contains catechins, an antioxidant that is thought to decrease high blood pressure. Because of the way matcha is prepared, it contains much more (some sources say more than 100 times more) catechins than other green teas, making it that much more effective. Research is currently being done on matcha's ability to protect against cancer.

Safety Considerations:
Matcha is generally regarded as safe.

Preparations:
Culinary ingredient, powdered, teas

TIP: With about one-sixth as much caffeine as coffee, there are no restrictions to the amount used.

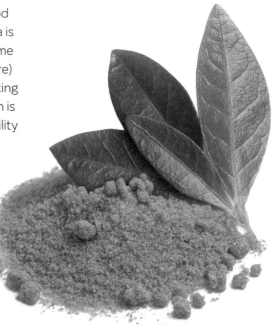

Milk Thistle

Latin Name: *Silybum marianum*
Common Name(s): Blessed milk thistle, holy thistle, Marian thistle, St. Mary's thistle

Vital Parts:
Seeds

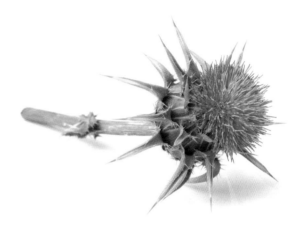

Medicinal Uses:
Milk thistle is often used for its protective and healing effects on the liver. It can also improve gallbladder function and help balance metabolism. Milk thistle can be used to treat chronic fatigue syndrome.

Safety Considerations:
Several human studies have demonstrated that milk thistle is safe, even when taken in substantial amounts. Despite this, individuals suffering from liver disease or undergoing cancer treatment should discuss use with a health-care professional before taking the herb. Those who are allergic to ragweed should stay away from this herb.

Preparations:
Standardized extract, teas

> **TIP:** Think twice before you decide to grow milk thistle in your garden, as it spreads rapidly and is very difficult to eradicate once established. If you want to grow milk thistle, just obtain some seeds, spread them on top of the soil, water, and watch for plants to emerge after several days. Harvest the tops after the flowers die back but before the wind carries the seeds away.

Mimosa

Latin Name: *Albizia julibrissin*
Common Name(s): Albizzia, tree of happiness, silk tree

Vital Parts:
Bark and flowers

Medicinal Uses:
When we look at plants and ask them what they have to offer us, mimosa is very clear. It brings back the light in our hearts and protects us from that which hurts us. Mimosa is ideal for addressing anxiety, depression, grief, insomnia, sore throat, blue or unstable moods, and swelling associated with trauma. There is nothing I've found like the combination of mimosa and holy basil (page 249) for easing the kind of intense, intractable sadness that has a presence of its own. The two together remind you that tomorrow is another day. Anxiety responds beautifully to the bark-heavy tincture or decoction.

Safety Considerations:
Not recommended during pregnancy.

Preparations:
Capsules, teas, tinctures

> **TIP:** The beautiful, fragrant pink flowers resemble puffs of tiny fiber-optic wires, and they glow from within. The leaves are sensitive and fold up when touched.

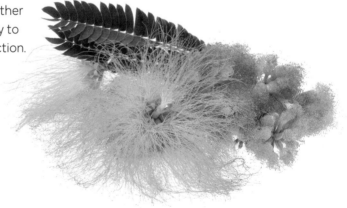

Mint

Latin Name: *Mentha* spp.
Common Name(s): Meadow tea

Vital Parts:
Leaves before bloom

Medicinal Uses:
Meadow tea is a spearmint (of which there are many), and the mild, soothing, and cooling flavor is something we all recognize. Peppermint, with a higher menthol content, is often used medicinally. Mint aids digestion and relieves nausea, gas, intestinal spasms, bloating, morning sickness, and inflammatory bowel conditions (such as intestinal virus, colitis, IBS, Crohn's disease, and diverticulitis). It also fights colds, flu, fever, and congestion; cools and relieves hot, itchy skin conditions, such as poison ivy and hives; and awakens the mind to aid in concentration.

Safety Considerations:
Peppermint can *increase* heartburn or reflux while spearmint *helps*. Note: I am *not* talking about the essential oil of mint here, as that is very concentrated and has completely different instructions! Much of the information out there is about the essential oil, and some recommend internal use. Consult with your doctor before taking essential oils internally.

Preparations:
Baths, culinary ingredient, syrups, teas, tinctures

TIP: A cup of spearmint tea after dinner aids digestion and may help with fatigue. A good cup of peppermint tea makes a head full of congestion feel better. Breathe in the steam while drinking.

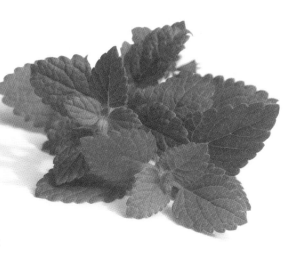

Monarda

Latin Name: *Monarda fistulosa, M. didyma, M. punctata*

Common Name(s): Bee balm, bergamot, horsemint, Oswego tea

Vital Parts:
Flowering tops

Medicinal Uses:
Monarda is used for digestive problems such as nausea, constipation, diarrhea, heartburn, stomachaches, and gas. It is soothing for respiratory ailments such as colds, flu, bronchitis, and other conditions that present with hot, spasmodic coughs. Monarda helps with chronic yeast infections that stem from leaky gut syndrome, as well as issues such as coughs, cystitis, urinary tract infections, sunburns, burns, and fevers. Monarda is one of the best herbs for reducing the symptoms of tinnitus, often with almost immediate effects. It can also be used as a wound wash to disinfect and encourage healing.

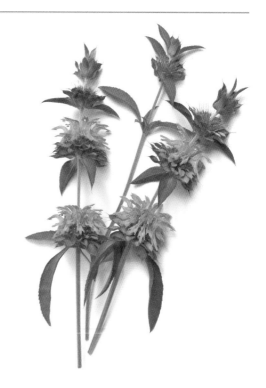

TIP: This is a great pollinator plant with a striking flower that makes a great addition to a garden. *M. fistulosa* flowers are a beautiful pale lavender color, and the *M. didyma* flowers are showstoppers in red or fuchsia.

Safety Considerations:
Monarda is generally regarded as safe.

Preparations:
Teas, tinctures, washes

Motherwort

Latin Name: *Leonurus cardiaca*
Common Name(s): Lionheart, lion's tail, mother's herb, mother's little helper

Vital Parts:
Flowering 6- to 8-inch tops, leaves, stems, and flowers

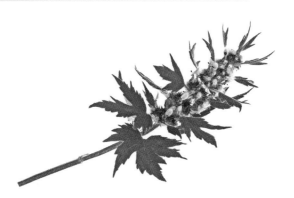

Medicinal Uses:
Motherwort supports the release of tension and irritation due to hormonal changes and premenstrual syndrome. It balances hormonal fluctuations for both young and elder people during the starting and ending of their menstrual cycles; helps calm hot flashes, night sweats, heart palpitations, insomnia, and depression during menopause; and can reduce stress during childbirth. Motherwort softens extreme emotional upset and helps improve healthy functioning of the male reproductive system, too. Motherwort also calms spasmodic conditions of the respiratory system, such as asthma.

Preparations:
Capsules, teas, tinctures

TIP: Be careful when harvesting the flowering tops—they are quite spiny! You may wish to use gardening gloves to hold the stalks while clipping them to protect yourself from any startling pokes.

Safety Considerations:
Motherwort is generally regarded as safe, but if you are on heart medications, consult with your doctor before using. People who are or might be pregnant should avoid motherwort because of its uterine stimulant action.

Mullein

Latin Name: *Verbascum thapsus*
Common Name(s): Aaron's rod, Adam's flannel, beggar's blanket, beggar's stalk, candlewick plant, clown's lungwort, common mullein, flannel leaf, golden rod, great mullein, hag's taper, Jupiter's staff, quaker rouge, shepherd's club, shepherd's staff, St. Peter's staff, torchwort, velvet dock

Vital Parts:
Leaves, flowers, roots

Medicinal Uses:
Mullein is useful as an antiviral and antibiotic, staving off illness. It also reduces inflammation of mucus membranes and calms muscle spasms, while also relieving pain. Mullein is also good for joint pain, both applied externally and taken internally. The warm flower oil is useful for hemorrhoids. Mullein promotes healing of wounds, cuts, and abrasions. When infused and warmed with a little garlic, it makes an effective ear drop for earaches and infections. The leaves have a long tradition as the main ingredient in smoking blends used for asthma and lingering coughs. It also helps relieve urinary issues and increase urine output.

Safety Considerations:
The fine hairs on this plant can irritate skin and mucus membranes, so be sure to strain preparations well.

Preparations:
Infused oil, poultices, teas, tinctures

TIP: The first-year plant is a basal rosette of fuzzy, pale blue-green leaves, and those are the roots to harvest for medicine. The leaves are always good to harvest. If you harvest the roots, be sure there are other plants around so you'll have more next year.

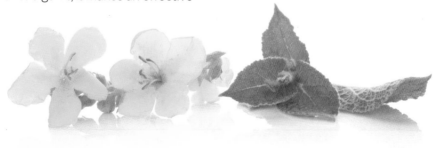

Nasturtium

Latin Name: *Tropaeolum* spp.
Common Name(s): Garden nasturtium, Indian cress

Vital Parts:
Leaves before the plant blooms

Medicinal Uses:
Nasturtium tea has a long history of use in stimulating the scalp and encouraging healthy hair growth. It is used to help heal wounds, including those that show infection and are slow to heal. The leaves contain carotenoids and flavonoids, valuable compounds that boost the immune system, making nasturtium another great herb to fight against sore throats, coughs, bronchitis, congestion, and colds. Bacterial and fungal infections such as candida, ringworm, and athlete's foot respond well to soaking in nasturtium-leaf tea or applied poultices. Nasturtium also has the surprising ability to relieve symptoms of seasonal allergies, like sneezing, runny nose, and dry, itchy eyes. It's been used historically for kidney problems and as a diuretic. For some, the tea helps with mild muscle pain.

Safety Considerations:
People who are or might be pregnant should avoid nasturtium. Additionally, it can cause contact dermatitis, so test a small area of skin before applying a poultice.

Preparations:
Culinary ingredient, poultices, rinses, teas, tinctures

TIP: Nasturtium seeds are very hot and spicy. They make a great little snack while working in the garden, or they can be grated and used like pepper or added to a spice blend for seasoning.

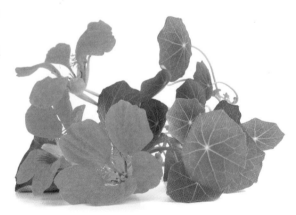

Oats

Latin Name: *Avena sativa*
Common Name(s): Common oats, milky oats, oatstraw, wild oats

Vital Parts:
Aerial parts

Medicinal Uses:
Oats are wonderful and skin-soothing when used in bathwater. When the whole plant is harvested and dried while green, including the seeds, it is called oatstraw. Oatstraw is a rejuvenating and restorative mineral tonic. Milky oats are the most commonly discussed form of oats. For just a few days, the unripe seeds excrete white, milky latex when squeezed, which can be used to feed and strengthen the nerves and their communication pathways. Milky oat tincture is the best way to access the herb's potential, and helps with adrenal exhaustion, difficulty concentrating, loss of libido, anxiety, depression, irritability, and postpartum blues. It is grounding, helping fortify people during grief, and promotes emotional well-being. Oatmeal is the ripe seed. It provides nourishment to the body and the skin while supporting the nervous system.

Safety Considerations:
Oats are generally regarded as safe.

Preparations:
Baths, culinary ingredient, tinctures

TIP: When the kernels begin to develop, be sure you have your alcohol ready to go in the house because it is only milky for about a week. Test for the milk (latex) every day by pinching one of the oats. When a small drop of white liquid appears, it is time to make tincture.

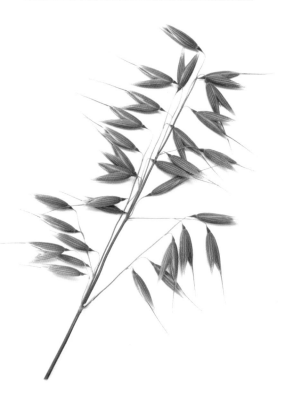

Onion

Latin Name: *Allium cepa*
Common Name(s): Bulb onion, common onion

Vital Parts:
Bulb

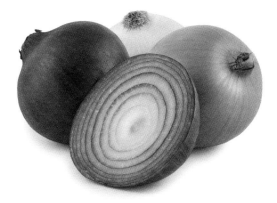

Medicinal Uses:

When eaten raw, onion prevents growth of *Helicobacter pylori*, which can cause ulcers. Onion can be applied externally as a poultice or plaster to wounds and sores. It draws out pus and infection, soothes inflammation, and calms lung spasms. Internally, an onion tincture can help with chronic bladder infections. Onion stimulates the circulatory system to reduce angina, arteriosclerosis, and heart attacks and eases coughs, colds, and flu.

Safety Considerations:

Onion is generally regarded as safe.

Preparations:

Culinary ingredient, plaster, poultice, tinctures

TIP: Plant onions in early spring in rows 4 to 6 inches apart by planting sets, root-side down, about 1 inch beneath the surface. Compost the soil and water it well. If starting with seeds, begin indoors either in the autumn or midwinter, as onions are a biennial and need a long growing season to develop a decent bulb. Weed thoroughly and mulch with grass clippings to avoid weeds choking out baby onions. Onions grown from sets can be harvested throughout the season, using early growth as scallions, then using the bulb further in the season once it matures. Harvest in late summer or early fall.

Oregano

Latin Name: *Origanum vulgare*
Common Name(s): Joy of the mountains, Spanish thyme, wild marjoram

Vital Parts:
Leaves, stems, flowers

Medicinal Uses:
Oregano is ideal for addressing coughs, colds, bronchitis and many other lung issues, acne, ringworm, athlete's foot, cramps, virus or flu, gingivitis, urinary tract infection, arthritis, digestion, and muscular aches and pains. Oregano can be very helpful with acne that's caused by bacteria by making a strong wash (tea) or a facial with the powdered herb, some clay, and witch hazel. The same can be done for ringworm, twice a day. When a virus starts flying around the office, some oregano tea can help keep the illness at bay.

Safety Considerations:
While the plant has been used medicinally for thousands of years, essential oil was not available to most people. The liquid, undiluted essential oil should be used by trained aromatherapists only. The essential oil is available in capsule form—follow label directions. Avoid the oil if pregnant.

Preparations:
Capsules, culinary ingredient, essential oils, liquids, teas, tinctures

TIP: Oregano is considered safe in the amounts that would be eaten, meaning that strong tea, or lots of extra oregano on that pizza, sub, salad, or any of the myriad dishes in which it shines are perfectly fine.

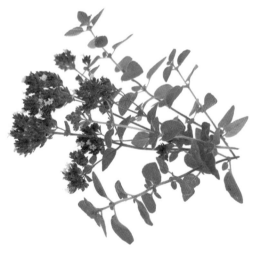

Parsley

Latin Name: *Petroselinum crispum*
Common Name(s): Garden parsley, parsley breakstone, petersylinge, rock parsley

Vital Parts:
Fresh or dried leaf

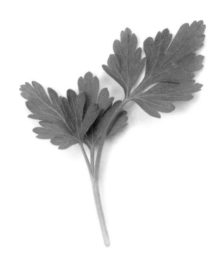

Medicinal Uses:
Parsley helps treat edema and poor fluid circulation in the legs, and can also stimulate kidney function. Parsley can be used as a food daily, if desired. It is extremely high in vitamin C. It is also high in vitamin K, which is supportive of bone health and essential for blood clotting, and vitamin A, which is important for the eyes. Chewing on a few parsley leaves will keep your breath smelling fresh.

TIP: Nutritive herbs are vitamin- and mineral-rich food sources. Drinking teas and vinegars infused with nutritive herbs is the best way to extract their minerals, such as calcium, magnesium, potassium, silica, zinc, and iron.

Safety Considerations:
Avoid during pregnancy in more than culinary servings, as it dries up breast milk. If you're on blood-thinning medication, check with your doctor before taking parsley medicinally.

Preparations:
Culinary ingredient, juices, teas

Passionflower

Latin Name: *Passiflora incarnata*
Common Name(s): Apricot vine, maypop, passion vine

Vital Parts:
Leaves, stems, flowers

Medicinal Uses:
Passionflower tea or tincture relaxes in several different ways. It is best known for stopping circular thinking, or when the brain goes over and over the same (usually unpleasant) thoughts. It is a hypnotic herb, meaning that it is quite strong, and it also relaxes muscles. Good night! Passionflower is surprisingly effective for nerve pain and shingles.

Safety Considerations:
Not for use in pregnancy or in conjunction with other relaxing or sedating medications. Not for use with MAOIs or blood thinners. Also avoid two to three weeks before surgery as it may increase the effects of anesthesia in the brain.

Preparations:
Capsules, pills, teas, tinctures

TIP: Passionflower is pretty easygoing when it comes to planting and doesn't really ask for much: some sunlight or partial shade, a warmish climate (though it's known to withstand zone-5 winter temps), and moist soil.

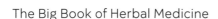

Peach

Latin Name: *Prunus persica*
Common Name(s): Nectarine, peacher-ine, Persian plum

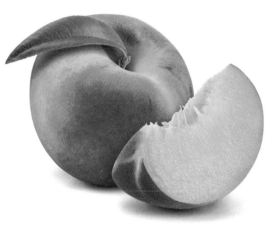

Vital Parts:
Leaf, bark, flower

Medicinal Uses:
Externally, peach soothes insect stings and the associated inflammation. Internally, it reduces digestive inflammation, eases nausea and vomiting, reduces diarrhea, and expels intestinal worms. Peach calms coughs from pertussis and other respiratory ailments, including dry, tickling coughs. It also stops nervous twitches and spasms, calms the immune system during allergic and asthmatic episodes, reduces anxiety and tension, and reduces feelings of burnout and insomnia.

Safety Considerations:
Peach is generally regarded as safe.

Preparations:
Compresses, culinary ingredient, infused oil, teas, tinctures

TIP: Take 30 drops of tincture 3 times a day or every 20 minutes for an acute episode (such as an insect sting) or 1 to 2 cups of tea daily. Increase up to 4 cups daily to expel worms. Apply compress of leaf tincture to insect stings and inflammation. Apply oil externally to inflammation and insect stings as needed.

Pennyroyal

Latin Name: *Mentha pulegium*
Common Name(s): Fleabane, mosquito plant, pennyrile, pudding grass, run-by-the-ground, tickweed

Vital Parts:
Flowering tops

Medicinal Uses:
Although pennyroyal has historically been used medicinally for several issues, since the late 1990s it has been shown to be too risky. Research shows that consumption of pennyroyal oil is linked to toxic liver injury and death. It was used for menstrual cramps and all sorts of menstrual issues, poor digestion, headaches, colds, coughs, and was used externally for a variety of skin issues and gout. The dried plant can be used in pet beds or where they spend time. It is often wrapped in bandanas and worn around a dog's neck as an insect deterrent, and sprigs can be worn in the hair or tucked in pockets while working in the garden. It is also a good ingredient in potpourri for a refreshing scent.

Safety Considerations:
Avoid any pennyroyal if pregnant or breastfeeding. Pennyroyal in any form should be used sparingly internally, if at all. It can cause liver, kidney, and nervous system damage. Do not give it to children.

Preparations:
Essential oils, teas

> **TIP:** There is no completely safe dosage. Pennyroyal essential oil should be used only by well-trained aromatherapists.

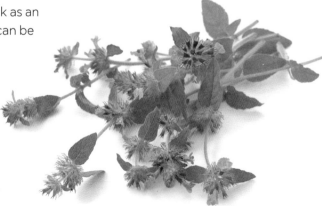

Pine

Latin Name: *Pinus* spp.
Common Name(s): Christmas tree, evergreen, tannenbaum

Vital Parts:
Needles, pollen, and pitch or sap

Medicinal Uses:
Pine eases inflammation and swelling of the upper- and lower-respiratory systems. The infusion of pine needle or sap in alcohol is a good disinfectant for wounds on skin, tissues, and membranes. Clearing away bacteria and all kinds of pathogens, pine speeds healing both inside and out. Pine teas and tinctures of needles or sap are thought to improve circulation and boost immunity. Salves made from the sap can be used on muscle and joint pain, and the inner bark can be made into a field dressing to keep wounds clean and germ-free.

Safety Considerations:
Pine pollen can cause allergic reactions even in those who aren't normally allergic to pine. I found this to be true the first time I gathered it.

Preparations:
Infused honey, infused oil, liniments, salves, teas, tinctures

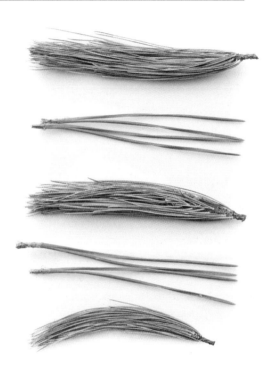

TIP: Gathering pine sap is dirty work. Be sure to wear clothes that you don't mind getting ruined. Take a sharp knife and a small wax paper–lined tin. Look for globs of sap where the bark has been injured, and peel off and place into your tin. You can also find small pearls of sap inside dropped cones.

Plantain

Latin Name: *Plantago* spp.

Common Name(s): Bird seed, common plantain, cuckoo's bread, devil's shoestring, dooryard plantain, Englishman's foot, healing blade, rabbit ears, rat-tail, ribwort, ripple grass, snakeweed, wagbread, waybread, waybroad

Vital Parts:
Leaves, seeds

Medicinal Uses:
Plantain is healing to the entire digestive system, beginning as a soothing gargle for mouth and gum irritations, then moving through the throat to calm soreness and into the esophagus where it can help relieve and soothe membranes that have been irritated with acid, and then into the stomach, where it is helpful in the case of ulcers. In the end, it goes on to soothe the entire system and relieve constipation, bladder inflammation, hemorrhoids, and even the kidneys. Psyllium is a specific variety of plantain, the seeds of which are used specifically for digestion and regularity. That same combination of astringency and mucilage is a boon for the respiratory tract, helping tighten, dry, and soothe. For the skin, it tackles insect bites, rashes, splinters, eczema, burns, and psoriasis.

Safety Considerations:
Plantain is generally regarded as safe for everyone, including infants and the elderly.

Preparations:
Face masks, oils, poultices, salves, soaks, spit poultices, teas, tinctures, tub teas, vinegars

> **TIP:** You can use teas or tinctures up to 3 times daily. External use is safe to repeat as needed.

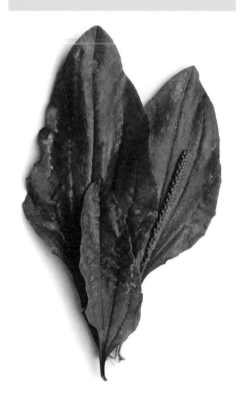

Raspberry

Latin Name: *Rubus idaeus*
Common Name(s): Framboise, rubi idaei folium, rubus

Vital Parts:
Leaf, root, fruit

Medicinal Uses:
Raspberry is widely known for its benefits in supporting pregnancy, labor, and delivery. Many cultures have used it to treat a wide range of ailments, including high blood pressure, kidney disorders, and infections. Raspberry also eases morning sickness, relieves sore throats, treats diarrhea, and reduces fever. Topically, its leaves are a powerful disinfectant and are applied to wounds to speed healing. They fight acne, shrink pores, and smooth skin texture. Raspberry is used as a natural SPF in moisturizers, creams, and oils.

Safety Considerations:
Raspberry is generally regarded as safe.

Preparations:
Compresses, culinary ingredient (fruit), oils, poultices, salves, teas, tinctures

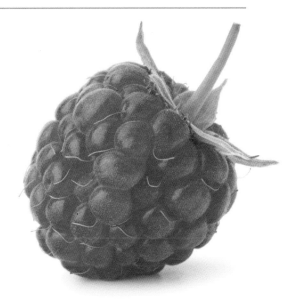

TIP: Raspberry bushes thrive in zones 3 to 9 in areas with full sun, fertile, well-drained soil, and good air circulation. Don't plant near an area that grows or used to grow tomatoes, potatoes, peppers, eggplants, bramble berries, or roses, which can leave behind harmful diseases that can attack and destroy the fruit.

Reishi Mushroom

Latin Name: *Ganoderma lucidum*
Common Name(s): Lingzhi (China), mannentake (Japan)

Vital Parts:
Fruiting body (mostly), spores, mycelium

Medicinal Uses:
Reishi mushroom is ideal for addressing infection, stress, mental sluggishness, high blood pressure, high cholesterol, difficulty sleeping, lack of energy, inflammation, and pain. Stimulating a vigorous and healthy immune response is one of the most common uses of reishi. Additionally, as an adaptogen, it may improve sleep and decrease the effects of stress, which also help support the immune system. In some Asian countries, it has been approved for use for a couple decades for cancer and is used in conjunction with chemotherapy.

Safety Considerations:
Avoid if you are pregnant, breastfeeding, about to have surgery, have any type of blood disorder, have high or low blood pressure, or take medication for diabetes. Reishi mushroom is very effective, so please check with your primary care physician if you are being treated for any condition before using it.

Preparations:
Capsules, dried whole, powdered, sliced, tinctures

TIP: Dosage depends on the type of preparation and condition it is addressing. As a preventive, many people drink it in tea as part of a blend once a day or more.

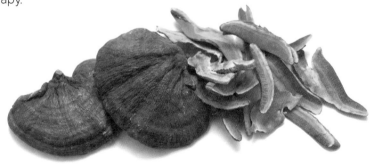

Rhodiola

Latin Name: *Rhodiola rosea*
Common Name(s): Arctic root, golden root, rose root

Vital Parts:
Root

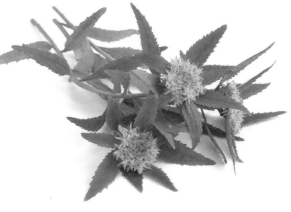

Medicinal Uses:
There are many pretty wild claims made about this sweet root, which is common with adaptogens, but this one had been approved for various uses in Russia and Sweden, meaning that their research has shown the herb to be capable of improving energy and neurological functions. Rhodiola is particularly useful for someone who pushes their physical endurance. It drastically reduces recovery time after a workout. Rhodiola is also ideal for addressing anxiety, depression, fatigue, headaches, lack of energy, mental fatigue, inability to concentrate, poor memory, stress, and general weakness.

Safety Considerations:
Avoid use if suffering from bipolar disorder. Consult your health-care provider before using if pregnant, nursing, or taking medication for emotional issues. Rhodiola is taken on an empty stomach earlier in the day so it doesn't keep you up. It can cause vivid dreams.

Preparations:
Capsules, tablets, teas, tinctures

TIP: Prepared as a tea, take 1 to 2 cups a day. As a tincture, 20 to 35 drops 1 or 2 times a day. Follow label directions on purchased products.

Rose

Latin Name: *Rosa* spp.
Common Name(s): Apothecary rose, beach rose, briar hip, briar rose, cabbage rose, damask rose, dogberry, eglantine gall, French rose, hep tree, hip fruit, hogseed, hop fruit, multiflora rose, sweet briar, wild rose, witches' briar

Vital Parts:
Whole flowers, petals

Medicinal Uses:
Rose reduces the pain, heat, and inflammation of burns (especially sunburn), wounds, scratches, abrasions, rashes, bites, and stings. Rose tincture quickly calms the system during any kind of upset, particularly in the case of trauma, like an accident or unexpected shock. It is believed to benefit cardiac health and blood pressure and improve poor circulation. Rose infusion strengthens bones and supports the endocrine system, helping people who menstruate maintain regularity and increasing fertility in others. Rose is also used for sore throats and mouth sores due to its astringency and moisturizing ability.

Safety Considerations:
No warnings other than possible allergy.

Preparations:
Compresses, essential oils, flower essences, infused honey, lotions, oils, poultices, rose water, soaps, teas, tinctures, vinegars

TIP: Fresh roses from florists are almost without fragrance, and they're typically grown with pesticides and preservatives. Grow your own or gather them in the wild. Once you've stuck your face in a basket of fresh, wild or homegrown rose petals, there will be no going back to anything less.

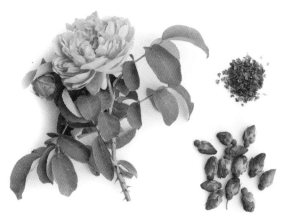

Rose Hips

Latin Name: *Rosa canina*
Common Name(s): Dog rose, hipberry, Persian rose, pink rose

Vital Parts:
Rose hips

Medicinal Uses:
Rose hips have 20 times more vitamin C than oranges. Whereas fresh rose hips are a major source of vitamin C, dried rose hips? Not so much. The act of drying the plant zaps a good bit of its C content. Rose hips can be used to treat osteoarthritis, rheumatoid arthritis, menstrual cramps, fever, infections, stomach issues like diarrhea, cramps, and irritation; reduce cholesterol; prevent and treat colds; and boost immunity. Externally, they can be used to replenish, repair, and protect skin; even skin tone; brighten skin; and improve elasticity.

Safety Considerations:
Although rose hips are considered safe, talk to your doctor before taking the herb as it may slow blood clotting, impact diabetes management, increase kidney stone risk, and impede the absorption of iron. Rose hips have small hairs inside the seed capsule, so avoid piercing or strain well if used for tea.

Preparations:
Compresses, essential oils, flower essences, infused honey, lotions, oils, poultices, rose water, soaps, teas, tinctures, vinegars

> **TIP:** Rose hips are the seed pods of the rose plant. Roses prefer light, sandy soil and loads of sunlight. Start with cuttings or seedlings and make some room for them to grow.

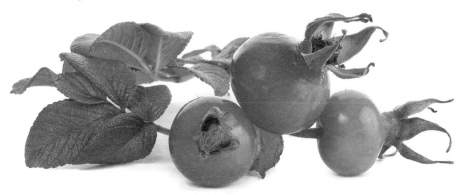

Rosemary

Latin Name: *Salvia rosmarinus,*
formerly Rosmarinus officinalis
Common Name(s): Compass plant,
compass-weed, dew of the sea, old man

Vital Parts:
Stems, leaves, flowers

Medicinal Uses:
Rosemary stimulates the brain as well
as the circulatory and nervous systems.
It improves peripheral circulation and
memory, making it especially useful for
individuals with Alzheimer's disease. It
also relieves headaches and migraines,
improves vision, and may help with
cataracts. As a tea, rosemary tones and
calms the digestive system, improves
digestion, stimulates bile production in
the gallbladder and the liver, reduces
fevers, relieves pain and sore muscles,
brings on menstruation, and reduces
high blood pressure. Externally, rosemary is used to relieve sciatica pain,
muscular pain, and neuralgia; decrease
dandruff; darken hair when used as a
hair rinse; prevent wrinkles; and ease
bruising, eczema, sprains, rheumatism,
and sore muscles. As a mouth freshener, rosemary freshens the breath
and soothes sore throats, gums, and
canker sores.

Safety Considerations:
Rosemary can interfere with some
medications, such as anticoagulants, blood pressure medications,
and diuretics.

Preparations:
Capsules, culinary ingredient, infused
oil, teas, tinctures, vinegars

TIP: A good whiff of rosemary stimulates your brain function and helps
wake you up. Rub it between your
hands to release the essential oil.

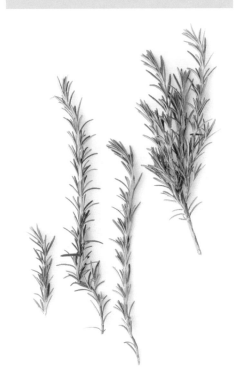

Sage

Latin Name: *Salvia officinalis,*
Salvia spp.
Common Name(s): Broadleaf sage,
clary sage, common sage, culinary
sage, dalmatian sage, garden sage,
golden sage, kitchen sage, purple sage,
smudge, tri-color sage, true sage

Vital Parts:
Leaves

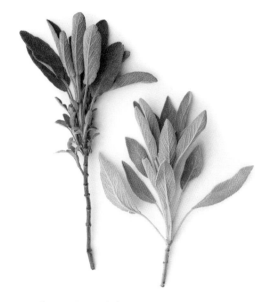

Medicinal Uses:
Internally, sage goes after excess
mucus, firms up membranes, and can
help with excessive perspiration or
saliva. Sage also helps dry up breast
milk when weaning children off breastfeeding. Sage helps with mouth, gum,
and throat issues. It is calming and
grounding when used either internally
or topically. It has been used traditionally to bring down fevers and promote
sleep. Menopausal hot flashes respond
well to sage tea or tincture. Sage has
been found to be capable of killing
E. coli. Sage tea with meals promotes
digestion and helps with stomach
pain, excess gas, diarrhea, bloating,
and heartburn.

Safety Considerations:
Avoid in pregnancy or
while breastfeeding.

Preparations:
Culinary ingredient, fresh, gar-
gles, mouthwash, smudge, teas,
tinctures, vinegars

TIP: Sage is very easy to grow. Check
with your garden nursery for hardiness
information in your region. Sage needs
good drainage, proper air circulation,
and plenty of sunshine. Even in the
middle of a cold winter I can typically
find some usable leaves.

Self-Heal

Latin Name: *Prunella*

Common Name(s): All-heal, blue curls, brownwort, carpenter's herb, heal-all, hock-heal, sicklewort, woundwort, xia ku cao

Vital Parts:
Flowers, leaves, and stems

Medicinal Uses:
The ingredient profile for self-heal contains cancer preventives, STD treatments, and antioxidants known to prevent and treat heart disease and boost immunity. It's also used to treat Crohn's disease, diarrhea, colic, gastroenteritis, throat issues, reduce fever, headache, liver disease, and muscle spasms. Used externally, self-heal fights inflammation and irritation, and tightens pores. From a psychological perspective, it's taken to boost mood, raise energy levels, and awaken self-confidence.

Safety Considerations:
Although no toxicity has been reported, herbalists suggest avoiding self-heal if you're pregnant or breastfeeding.

Preparations:
Eye wash, mouthwash, oils, ointments, salves, soaps, splashes

TIP: Like many herbs with weed-like sensibilities, self-heal can grow just about anywhere, but it thrives in woods, meadows, and forest environments. Partial sun and mild temperatures are its sweet spot. If you're in a space with wet conditions, this herb spreads like wildfire.

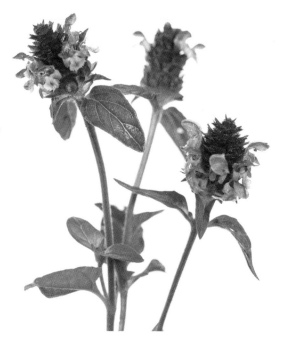

Shatavari

Latin Name: *Asparagus racemosus*
Common Name(s): Buttermilk toot, climbing asparagus, queen of herbs, satavar, satavari, shatamull, tien men dong, wild asparagus

Vital Parts:
Root

Medicinal Uses:
Shatavari is ideal for addressing stress, cough, diarrhea, depression, aging skin (collagen breakdown), mood swings, infertility, low weight, high blood pressure, gastric ulcers, weakness, inability to concentrate, and depression. Symptoms of menopause are often helped with shatavari, cooling the body during hot flashes, calming the mind, increasing mental acuity, and helping with sleep. In many cases, it may help PMS by relieving pain and bloating, improving sleep, and cooling those mood swings. Shatavari is thought to help reduce the incidence of kidney stones by blocking the production of oxalates and increasing magnesium in the blood.

Safety Considerations:
Do not use if allergic to asparagus. May cause weight gain.

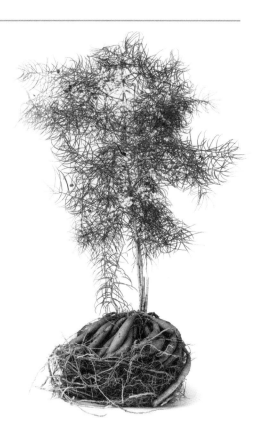

Preparations:
Capsules, powders (sometimes referred to as shatavari churna) mixed with milk, ghee, or water, tablets, tinctures

TIP: The recommended dosage is up to 500 mg powdered or as a capsule twice daily, or 25 to 30 drops of tincture 2 to 3 times a day.

Skullcap

Latin Name: *Scutellaria lateriflora*
Common Name(s): Helmet flower, hoodwort, mad dog skullcap, mad dog weed

Vital Parts:
Aerial parts

Medicinal Uses:
Skullcap is great when you need to relax or get past some nervous tension or anxiety but still want to get things done. It's ideal for addressing anxiety, nervous headaches, indigestion, insomnia, nervousness, muscle cramps, pain, panic attacks, and stress. A nice cup of tea or some tincture provides quick relief.

Safety Considerations:
Do not use in pregnancy or during breastfeeding. There are varying opinions on whether overuse causes liver damage, so err on the side of caution. Do not overuse; follow directions for use on package.

Preparations:
Capsules, teas, tinctures

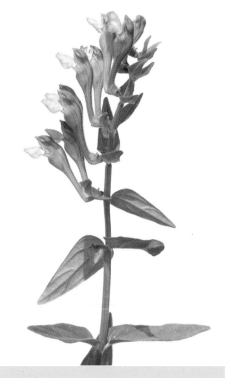

TIP: Prepared as a tea, take 1 cup of skullcap 3 times a day. As a tincture, take 40 to 80 drops up to 3 times a day. For capsules, follow directions on the manufacturer's label.

Slippery Elm

Latin Name: *Ulmus rubra*
Common Name(s): Indian elm, moose elm, orme, red elm, sweet elm

Vital Parts:
Inner bark and wood

Medicinal Uses:
A tea of slippery elm is used to treat cough, sore throats, and laryngitis; eases digestive and gastrointestinal problems like constipation, diarrhea, IBS, ulcers, and hemorrhoids. It heals skin conditions like burns, cold sores, boils, ulcers, abscesses, and wounds, and eases tooth pain. Used externally, slippery elm soothes aging skin, combats wrinkles, and erases sun damage.

Safety Considerations:
Don't take slippery elm if you're breast-feeding or pregnant. It's rumored to cause miscarriages. In some instances, slippery elm can cause an allergic reaction. If skin gets irritated, discontinue use or lower the dose.

Preparations:
Compresses, lozenges, poultices, teas

TIP: You'll find slippery elm in places with poorly drained soil like riverbeds, stream banks, lowlands, mountain bottoms, or canyons. It's best suited for environments that allow for the tree to have moist soil and partial sunlight.

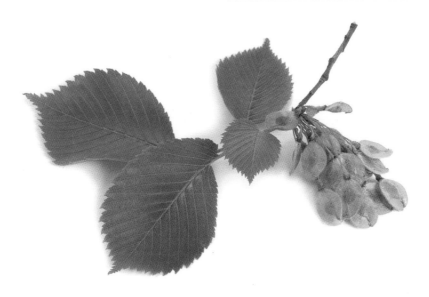

Stinging Nettles

Latin Name: *Urtica dioica*
Common Name(s): Burn hazel, nettles

Vital Parts:
Leaves, roots

Medicinal Uses:
An astringent and antibacterial, nettle soothes eczema while fighting allergic responses. Nettle holds a lifetime of benefits. It evens out hormones and alleviates PMS symptoms, helps with excessive bleeding, supports nursing people with milk production, and, finally, helps people through and beyond menopause by supporting the adrenals and the endocrine system. Some believe that the stings interfere with the way the body transmits pain signals by temporarily wearing out the "transmitter" so that pain signals aren't received. The sting is sometimes intentionally administered in a process called urtification on painful joints caused by osteoarthritis or rheumatoid arthritis. The tea is effective as a pain reliever and can be used in combination with an external application.

Safety Considerations:
Those taking blood-thinning, blood pressure, or diuretic medications should avoid nettles, as they may amplify the effects of the pharmaceuticals.

Preparations:
Capsules, creams, hair care products, nourishing herbal infusions, pills, salves, teas, tinctures, vinegars

TIP: I planted one small nettle plant 3 years ago. It is now a 6-foot-round plot, growing by the day. I strongly suggest using raised beds or sinking a metal barrier into the soil to contain nettles.

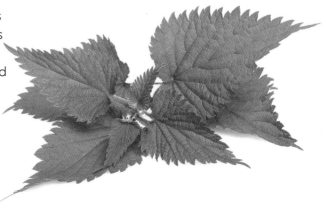

St. John's Wort

Latin Name: *Hypericum perforatum*
Common Name(s): Chase-devil, goatweed, klamath weed, St. Joan's wort

Vital Parts:
Flowering tops, top 6 inches or so

Medicinal Uses:
When applied topically, St. John's wort can work as a sunscreen and for sunburn relief. As a tincture, it relieves anxiety, depression, and seasonal affective disorder (SAD) and improves sleep quality. It can also suppress viruses such as chicken pox, herpes, and shingles. A tincture taken in the evening reduces bedwetting in children. The infused oil relieves muscle cramps such as charley horses, sciatic nerve pain, and other nerve conditions. It also improves fungal issues such as candida, thrush, athlete's foot, and ringworm. St. John's wort may heal wounds and reduce nerve damage when applied topically.

Safety Considerations:
Should not be taken in conjunction with certain medications, especially antidepressant or antianxiety medicines but also contraceptives, blood thinners, antibiotics, and others. Check with your doctor if you're using prescribed medications. May increase sun sensitivity.

Preparations:
Capsules, infused oil, pills, teas, tinctures

TIP: Prepared as a tea, take 1 cup of St. John's wort 3 times a day. As a tincture, take 25 to 50 drops up to 3 times a day. For pills and capsules, follow the directions on the manufacturer's label.

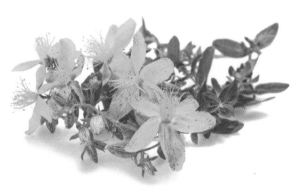

Tea Tree

Latin Name: *Melaleuca alternifolia*
Common Name(s): Narrow-leaved paperbark, narrow-leaved tea-tree

Vital Parts:
Leaves

Medicinal Uses:
Tea tree oil is a popular herbal medicine that helps with skin issues, including acne, dandruff, minor wounds, and infections. Used as a cream and applied twice a day for one month, it can also treat athlete's foot.

Safety Considerations:
Tea tree essential oil and products containing tea tree should not be taken internally. Some people with sensitive skin develop contact dermatitis, itching, or allergic reactions when tea tree oil and products containing it are applied externally.

Preparations:
Creams, essential oils, ointments, salves

TIP: As tea tree products are popular, it is not at all difficult to locate them. You'll find them at major retailers, health-food stores, and online. Potted tea trees are sometimes available at nurseries (not to be confused with ti plants/trees) and may be grown indoors in cold climates. They require rich soil and plenty of moisture to flourish.

Thyme

Latin Name: *Thymus vulgaris*
Common Name(s): Common thyme, creeping thyme, garden thyme, mother of thyme, mountain thyme, wild thyme

Vital Parts:
Leaves

Medicinal Uses:
Thyme is very valuable in compresses, salves, or washes for acne, scalp problems, rashes, bites, wounds, or parasites, such as scabies and lice. As an antifungal, thyme offers relief from athlete's foot or jock itch. Syrup or tea made from thyme will break up and move excess mucus in chest colds or stuffy heads, while putting the brakes on viral infections. Thyme can help calm coughs and bronchitis and soothe sore throats while encouraging restful sleep. Like so many aromatic culinary herbs, thyme is great for the digestive tract, improving appetite, relieving excess gas, and aiding the absorption of nutrition. As a tea during PMS, the diuretic, anti-inflammatory, and antispasmodic properties are marvelous and carry through during menses to relieve cramps, pain, and insomnia.

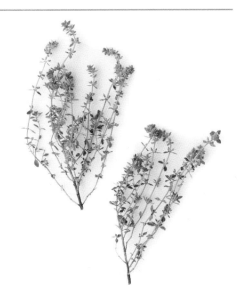

Safety Considerations:
Thyme contains thymol, so large quantities (generally referring to the use of essential oil) used over an extended period may cause damage to the heart, lungs, kidneys, liver, and nervous system. Never take thyme essential oil internally or use it undiluted on the skin.

Preparations:
Compresses, culinary ingredient, essential oils, poultices, salves, syrups, teas, tinctures, vinegars, washes

TIP: Prepared as a tea or tincture, take 3 times a day. Culinary use to taste is unlimited (within reason).

Turmeric

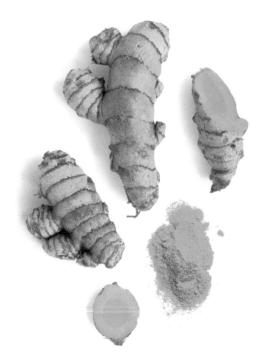

Latin Name: *Curcuma longa*
Common Name(s): Common turmeric, curcumin, haldi, Indian saffron, turmeric root, wild curcuma

Vital Parts:
Rhizomes

Medicinal Uses:
Turmeric is a powerful anti-inflammatory and, as such, can be used to alleviate arthritis, osteoarthritis, rheumatism, inflammatory bowel disease, and muscle aches. It can help combat atherosclerosis, regulate blood pressure, and assist with blood clotting. Historically it was used to treat joint pain as well as skin, respiratory, and digestive issues.

Safety Considerations:
Turmeric increases bile production and may cause heartburn to worsen. It should be used sparingly by those who suffer from gastric reflux.

Preparations:
Capsules, culinary ingredient, standardized extract, teas

TIP: A culinary staple in many areas, turmeric is widely available in supermarkets, at major retailers, at health-food stores, and online.

Uva Ursi

Latin Name: *Arctostaphylos uva-ursi*
Common Name(s): Bearberry, kinni-kinnick, pinemat manzanita

Vital Parts:
Leaves

Medicinal Uses:
Uva ursi has a history of being used to treat urinary tract infections (UTIs) and bladder infections (page 237). Uva ursi can also alleviate bronchitis as well as constipation. It can also be used externally as an antiseptic to clean minor cuts and scrapes.

Safety Considerations:
People who are pregnant or nursing should not use uva ursi. The herb contains hydroquinone, a compound that can cause liver damage if taken long-term; do not take it for more than two weeks at a time. Do not take uva ursi if you have liver or kidney disease.

Preparations:
Capsules, creams, ointments, salves, teas, tinctures

TIP: The best way to grow this herb is to purchase young shrubs and transplant them into your herb garden or to grow new shrubs from cuttings that have been dipped in rooting hormone. Uva ursi does best in gravelly soil with a pH of 5 or less. It prefers full sun and thrives in cool climates; it is hardy to −50°F.

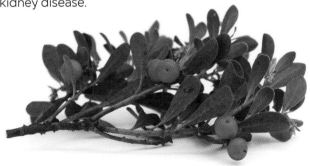

Valerian

Latin Name: *Valeriana officinalis*
Common Name(s): All-heal, common valerian, garden heliotrope

Vital Parts:
Roots, leaves, flowers

Medicinal Uses:
Valerian most often comes to mind for trouble sleeping. It is also ideal for addressing anxiety, dizziness, muscle tension, muscular spasms, menstrual cramps, menopause symptoms, nervous tension, and palpitations. If you can find tincture or tea made with valerian flowers, they have a gentler action, and I like them because they relax me rather than jazzing me up like the roots.

Safety Considerations:
Valerian is a powerful sedative. Do not take it before driving, operating machinery, or conducting tasks that require close attention. Valerian can increase the sedative effects of substances such as sleep aids and alcohol. Some individuals exhibit an idiosyncratic reaction to the herb, exhibiting wakefulness and excitability after taking it.

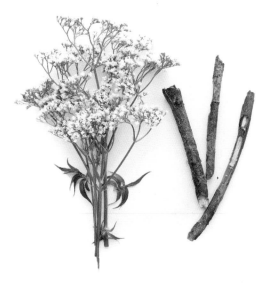

Preparations:
Capsules, powders, teas, tinctures

TIP: This perennial loves moist, rich soil and partial shade. Another self-sower, once you plant valerian, you'll likely find it in abundance everywhere in your garden.

Willow

Latin Name: *Salix* spp.
Common Name(s): Basket willow, black willow, crack willow, purple willow, pussy willow, white willow

Vital Parts:
Leaf, twig, inner bark

Medicinal Uses:
Willow is used to ease aches and pains, muscle spasms, inflammation, rheumatism, arthritis, gout, back pain, headaches, and neuralgia. It also helps reduce stomachaches, helps lower fevers, and relieves nervous insomnia.

Safety Considerations:
Use with caution if pregnant. Those on blood thinners or with hemophilia should avoid willow. Do not give to children with a viral infection with headaches. Use with caution if you are allergic to aspirin.

Preparations:
Capsules, standardized extract, teas

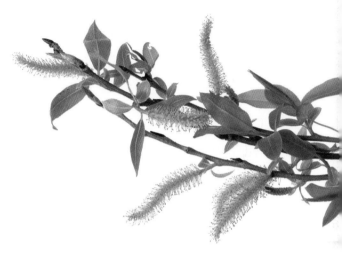

TIP: Willow prefers to grow in places where its roots have continuous access to water, so it is often found growing near streams, riverbanks, ponds, lakes, and other bodies of fresh water or in low-lying areas where water pools after rain. Harvest the leaves in spring and summer and the inner bark or twigs in spring or fall when the sap is rising or falling.

Wintergreen

Latin Name: *Gaultheria procumbens*
Common Name(s): Checkerberry, dewberry, ground holly, teaberry, woodsman's tea

Vital Parts:
Leaves and berries

Medicinal Uses:
Arthritis and muscular aches and pains respond well to wintergreen-infused massage oil or liniment. Wintergreen tea can settle a nervous stomach. The tea can assist with respiratory issues. I was asked years ago to provide a tea for a woman whose physician advised her to drink a tea that was half ephedra (now unfortunately banned due to overuse as a stimulant) and half wintergreen, for asthma, and she found that she rarely used her inhaler when she had the tea.

Safety Considerations:
Wintergreen essential oil is considered a toxin. It should be used only by trained aromatherapists. Those allergic to aspirin, or children with the flu or chicken pox, should not use wintergreen. Do not take in conjunction with anticoagulant medication. Not recommended during pregnancy.

Preparations:
Essential oils, liniments, ointments, teas

TIP: Use the tea or external application up to 3 times daily, not exceeding 2 weeks.

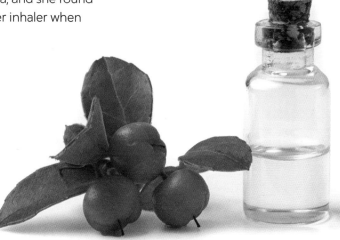

Witch Hazel

Latin Name: *Hamamelis virginiana*
Common Name(s): Snapping hazel, winterbloom

Vital Parts:
Leaves and bark

Medicinal Uses:
Witch hazel is used to soothe itching, irritating, and painful skin conditions, including diaper rash, insect stings and bites, eczema, and hemorrhoids. It also reduces swelling, bruises, varicose veins, and under-eye bags and dark circles. Witch hazel relieves colds, fever, varicose veins, and bruises. It treats damaged gums, swimmer's ear, and sore throats; eases cramping and discomfort from menstruation; and alleviates diarrhea.

Safety Considerations:
Avoid using if skin is sunburned, dry, overly sensitive, or windburned. Witch hazel is typically used externally, as the tannins it contains can cause serious indigestion in some individuals. If drinking witch hazel tea for a condition such as diarrhea or a urinary tract infection, take it for no longer than three days at a time.

Preparations:
Creams, decoctions, distillates, ointments, salves, teas

TIP: Witch hazel shrubs are massive in both size and flower output. With gorgeous yellow flowers, ripe fruits, and burgeoning buds—often blooming at the same time—it's found quite often in forests or woodsy areas. Adaptable to sunlight and soil types, it's loved by herbalists and gardeners because of its color and sweet aroma.

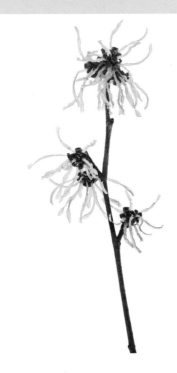

Woodruff

Latin Name: *Galium odoratum*
Common Name(s): Master of the woods, sweet-scented bedstraw, sweet woodruff, waldmeister

Vital Parts:
Leaves and flowers

Medicinal Uses:
Woodruff is ideal for addressing kidney and liver issues, circulatory problems and venous insufficiency, cramps, anxiety, arthritis, and constipation. The anti-inflammatory, antibiotic, and analgesic properties make woodruff a good traditional remedy for wounds and skin conditions. A tea made with woodruff is used for insomnia or restlessness. One of the most outstanding qualities is the sweet vanilla scent that intensifies as the plant dries, making it an excellent addition to scented pillows or potpourri. The most common use for woodruff in modern times involves adding flowering sprigs to Riesling or other sweet wine and serving it at May Day celebrations as a spring tonic.

Safety Considerations:
Large quantities or overuse can damage the liver. Do not use in conjunction with anticoagulant medications, including NSAIDS.

Preparations:
Compresses, dried, poultices, teas, washes

> **TIP:** There is no clear, official dosage. Please use in moderation.

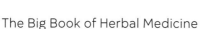

Yarrow

Latin Name: *Achillea millefolium*
Common Name(s): Bloodwort, carpenter's weed, death flower, devil's nettle, devil's plaything, field hoop, milfoil, nosebleed, old man's pepper, soldier's woundwort, staunchweed, thousand leaf, woundwort, yarroway

Vital Parts:
Aerial parts

Medicinal Uses:
Yarrow eases anxiety and stress and helps relieve insomnia. It also relieves pain and many stomach problems, including nausea, vomiting, gas, bloating, cramps, and diarrhea. The astringency of yarrow makes it brilliant at tightening and healing sore or bleeding gums and toning mucus membranes. People have long used yarrow internally for heavy bleeding due to uterine fibroids, endometriosis, ovarian cysts, or very heavy periods. Conversely, yarrow can also be used to stimulate menstruation and relieve menopausal night sweats. Yarrow is useful in reducing fevers by encouraging a sweat. It assists in fighting bacteria and infections, acts as a decongestant to ease coughs and sinus infections, and is anti-inflammatory. Yarrow is helpful for seasonal allergies and soothes hives and skin rashes.

Safety Considerations:
Individuals with clotting disorders should use caution with internal use of yarrow. Avoid yarrow in pregnancy. Fresh yarrow plant may (in rare cases) cause dermatitis, and some people are allergic to yarrow.

Preparations:
Baths, poultices, salves, sitz baths, teas, tinctures

TIP: Teas are a great way to use yarrow. Try blending it with echinacea, elderflower, ginger, and peppermint for colds, fevers, and flu-like symptoms. Try it with chamomile, linden, and catnip for restful sleep.

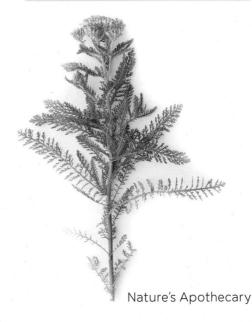

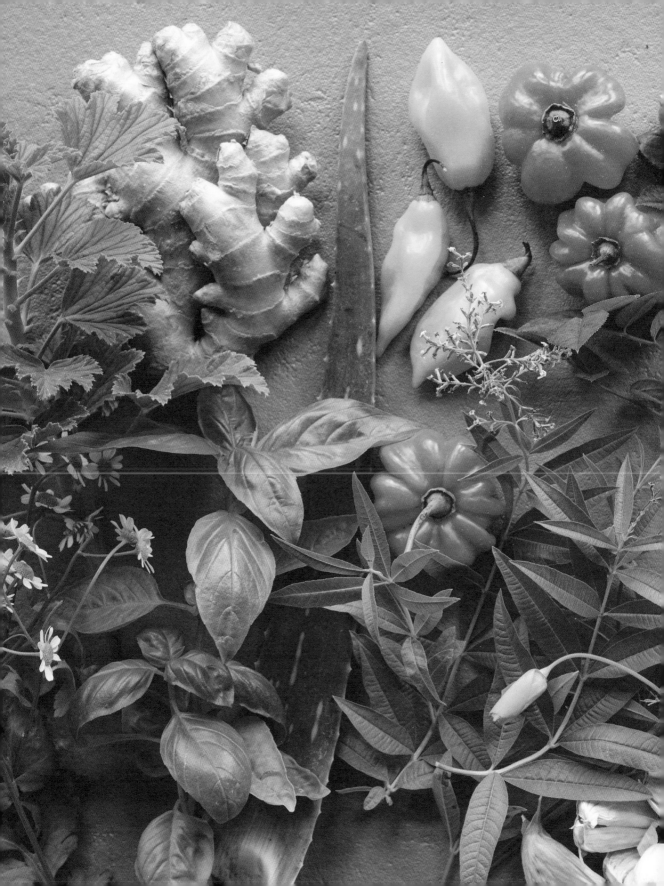

PART THREE

300 Remedies for Health and Wellness

Now that you understand the hows and whys of herbal medicine and have learned about 90 excellent plants, 300 remedies await! My favorite evening activity includes gathering some leaves or roots, and either immediately dunking them in alcohol or oil or prepping them to dry or freeze. I must warn you: This can be habit-forming—but it's fun!

The remedies are divided into chapters of physical issues, emotional issues, and skincare. Within each chapter, those remedies are listed alphabetically by ailment so they're easy to find.

However, you might notice that there is some overlap throughout the chapters. For example, taking care of the mind is taking care of the body, and taking care of the body and mind has benefits for the skin. It's all related.

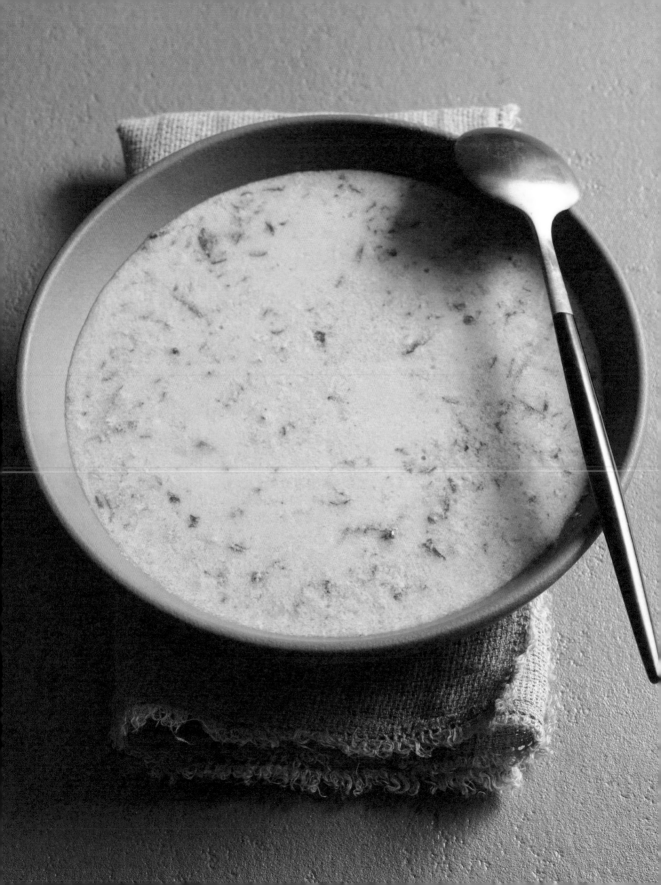

CHAPTER FIVE

Remedies for Physical Ailments

This is the point of introduction for many people getting started with medicinal herbs. Often a friend shares a simple remedy, which presents the healing power of herbs, and the journey begins.

The things you really need may already be in your kitchen. Others are in the yard, market, herb shop, health-food store, or online. Gathering them is half the fun! And then, suddenly, you're ready when a child is queasy in the middle of the night, or your partner has developed a hacking cough. Not only can you learn to help yourself, but herbs can help you on your quest to help your loved ones when they need it, too.

Cayenne Salve

The heat from the peppers and the ginger in this salve promotes circulation to speed healing while relieving pain. The peppermint oil is cooling and analgesic, making the combination very effective.

MAKES 12 TO 14 OUNCES

2 cups olive oil

½ cup red pepper flakes

1 tablespoon grated fresh ginger

2 ounces beeswax

1 teaspoon peppermint essential oil

1. In a slow cooker on low, infuse the olive oil with the pepper flakes and ginger for 4 to 6 hours.

2. Strain into a glass measuring cup or other container with a pouring lip. Compost the solids.

3. While the oil is still hot, stir in the beeswax until it melts.

4. Add the essential oil just before pouring the salve into labeled and dated jars. Store in a cool, dark place and use within 6 to 9 months.

5. To use, apply the cooled salve directly to the skin using an ice pop stick or the back of a clean spoon (this keeps bacteria from being introduced into the jar).

Barn Cat Balm

This salve works similarly to the popular brand Tiger Balm. It can be applied to sore, achy muscles and will help relieve the pain. It works for any type of muscle aches, including menstrual cramps, pulled or strained muscles, back pain, and sore post-garden-workout muscles.

CONTINUED »

MAKES 4 OUNCES

2 tablespoons
dried rosemary
2 tablespoons
dried peppermint
1½ tablespoons chopped
dried willow bark
1½ tablespoons
dried basil
1 tablespoon chopped
dried (cut and sifted)
mullein roots
1½ cups olive oil
1½ ounces beeswax

1. Follow the instructions in chapter 3 for making an herb-infused oil (page 30) and a salve (page 31), using the rosemary, peppermint, willow bark, basil, mullein, olive oil, and beeswax.

2. Label your salve with the name, ingredient list, and date it was made. Store in a cool, dark place and use within 6 to 9 months.

3. Apply a small amount of salve to affected muscles and massage into the area. Repeat as needed. You may find that applying heat can help increase the effect of the salve.

ACID REFLUX, NAUSEA, AND HEARTBURN

Fresh Ginger Tea

Tea made with fresh ginger is a simple yet effective remedy for acid reflux, nausea, and heartburn. It is safe to take during pregnancy and helps with morning sickness.

MAKES 1 DOSE

1 cup water
1 (2-inch) piece
fresh ginger
Raw honey or stevia, for
sweetening (optional)

1. Boil the water. While the water is heating, peel the ginger and slice it as thinly as possible. Place the ginger in a mug or teapot.

2. Add the boiling water, cover the mug or teapot, and allow the ginger to steep until the tea has cooled enough to drink. Sweeten the tea with a small amount of honey (if using).

3. Drink up to 3 cups a day.

Elderflower Tea

Drinking medicinal tea can be a useful ritual to incorporate into your healing routine. Elderflower is the white blossom of the elder tree. This flower has amazing anti-inflammatory and antiseptic properties that can calm the nerves and heal problems with the sinuses, eyes, lungs, and respiratory system. It's commonly used for colds and flu, sinus infections, and other respiratory issues. This herb can be very effective at alleviating allergy symptoms and boosting the immune system. Its delicate flavor also combines nicely with other herbs.

MAKES 2 CUPS

2 cups water
2 teaspoons dried elderflower

1. In a small saucepan, boil the water.

2. Drop the elderflower into the boiling water and remove the pan from the heat.

3. Allow the elderflower to steep in the water for 5 to 10 minutes. The longer it steeps, the stronger and more potent the tea will be.

4. Strain and drink it warm or add ice to make iced tea.

Nettle Infusion

To make a hot herbal tea infusion, you need to buy loose-leaf tea. Hot herbal tea infusions use a larger amount of herbs and are steeped for several hours so the vitamins and enzymes are fully drawn out. The longer the tea is steeped, the more nutrients it provides.

CONTINUED »

MAKES 4 CUPS

1 quart water
3 tablespoons
   dried nettles

1. Boil the water.

2. Place the nettles in a mason jar, then fill the jar to the top with the water. Cover with a lid, label, and date the jar.

3. Let the infusion steep for at least 1 hour. (To maximize the extraction of minerals from the nettles, steep longer—up to 24 hours.)

4. Strain and drink right away or store in the refrigerator for up to 3 days. Compost the solids.

ALLERGIES

Peppermint Facial Spa

Though the best way to treat seasonal allergies is to avoid known allergens as much as possible, it can be difficult to avoid occasional stuffy noses, teary eyes, and sneezing. When allergies attack, try this peppermint facial spa, and follow it up with a cup of hot peppermint tea. Peppermint is an excellent decongestant, and it helps reduce inflammation, bringing the relief you long for.

MAKES 1 DOSE

4 cups boiling water
6 drops peppermint
   essential oil

1. Place a large, sturdy bowl on a towel. Place a second towel and a box of tissues next to the bowl.

2. Pour the boiling water into the bowl and add the peppermint essential oil.

3. Sit in a chair with your face over the bowl. Drape the second towel over the back of your head and neck and let in fall down around the outside of the bowl, making a tent to trap the steam.

CONTINUED »

4. Close your eyes and breathe deeply. Use the tissues to blow your nose as needed.

5. Try to make the treatment last for at least 15 minutes. This facial can be repeated as often as necessary.

ALLERGIES

Pineapple Turmeric Juice

Bromelain is an enzyme found in the core and flesh of pineapples. It is a natural remedy for inflammation and can help reduce allergies, thanks to its anti-inflammatory and anti-allergic properties. Quercetin is a natural antioxidant and antihistamine and can be very helpful in relieving allergy symptoms. This antioxidant is a natural compound found in plant food such as citrus fruits, turmeric, apples, cranberries, dark berries, kale, and watercress, and its anti-inflammatory properties can help reduce redness and itchy eyes.

MAKES 2 SERVINGS

1 pineapple, peeled and
   cut into large chunks
2 oranges, cut into
   large slices
1 apple, cut into
   large slices
1 lemon, cut into
   large slices
1 (2-inch) piece
   unpeeled turmeric
   root, or 1 tablespoon
   ground turmeric
1 to 2 tablespoons
   raw honey

1. Run the fruits through a juicer to extract the juice.

2. Run the turmeric root through the juicer.

3. Add the honey to the juice and gently stir.

4. Drink one serving immediately, then label and date the bottle, and refrigerate the rest of the juice for up to 2 days.

Pain Relief Blend

Essential oils are often used for their mild anesthetic properties, which can help relieve localized pain. Oils such as cypress, sweet marjoram, peppermint, and ginger can work on the body in a similar way to nonsteroidal anti-inflammatory drugs, such as ibuprofen, by inhibiting the enzymes in the body that cause inflammation, pain, and swelling.

MAKES ⅓ OUNCE

2 drops cypress
   essential oil
2 drops sweet marjoram
   essential oil
2 drops ylang-ylang
   essential oil
2 drops peppermint
   essential oil

2 drops black pepper
   essential oil
2 drops ginger
   essential oil

10 mL glass bottle
   filled with almond oil,
   coconut oil, or other
   carrier oil of choice

Put the cypress, marjoram, ylang-ylang, peppermint, pepper, and ginger essential oils into the bottle of almond oil. Cover and shake the labeled bottle well. Apply a few drops and massage into your skin to relieve pain. Label and date the bottle, store it in a cool, dry place, and use it within 1 year.

Red Pepper Liniment

Hot red peppers contain capsaicin, a compound that stimulates blood flow, therefore easing the pain associated with arthritis, osteoarthritis, and rheumatism. This liniment is also effective for soothing bruises and sore muscles.

MAKES 20 TO 40 DOSES

5 tablespoons
   coconut oil

1 tablespoon very thinly
   sliced fresh cayenne
   chile (allowed to wilt

overnight to lose
moisture content)

CONTINUED »

1. In a small saucepan, melt the coconut oil over low heat. Stir in the cayenne chile and heat gently for 2 hours.

2. Strain the oil well. Compost the solids.

3. Pour the infused oil into a small labeled jar; let it cool completely before securing the lid. Store in a cool, dry place for up to 1 year.

4. Apply ½ teaspoon of the ointment at a time, up to 3 times a day, as needed. Wash your hands thoroughly after application. Avoid contact with eyes and mucous membranes.

ARTHRITIS

Turmeric Paste and Golden Milk

This is a classic Ayurveda turmeric paste that can be used to make golden milk, a warm, healing beverage with anti-inflammatory and antioxidant benefits. Golden milk originated in India and has been used to support the body and mind. In today's busy world, creating this recipe may take a bit of time. So, it's a good idea to make the paste in advance. You can also purchase the paste at a health-food store or online. It's traditionally made by mixing turmeric and ghee, and it can be stored in the refrigerator until you're ready to make the golden milk. Turmeric can help reduce pain and swelling in arthritis patients, and cloves contain eugenol, an anti-inflammatory chemical that interferes with the process that triggers arthritis pain.

MAKES 48 SERVINGS OF TURMERIC PASTE (2 TEASPOONS OF PASTE PER CUP OF MILK)

For the turmeric paste

½ cup ground turmeric

1 to 1½ cups water, plus more as needed

CONTINUED »

¼ teaspoon freshly
   ground black pepper
2 teaspoons
   ground cinnamon
2 teaspoons
   ground cardamom
1½ teaspoons
   ground ginger
½ teaspoon
   ground cloves
1 teaspoon
   ground nutmeg
Pinch Himalayan salt
½ cup ghee or coconut
   oil (as a vegan option)

For the golden milk

1 cup coconut milk or
   nut milk of choice
2 teaspoons
   turmeric paste
Raw honey, coconut
   sugar, stevia, or other
   sweetener of choice,
   for sweetening

To make the turmeric paste

1. Put the ground turmeric and water in a small saucepan over medium-low heat, stirring constantly. Keep stirring for a few minutes until the mixture has reached a paste-like consistency. (Use more or less water depending on how thin or thick you prefer the paste.)

2. Slowly stir in the pepper, cinnamon, cardamom, ginger, cloves, nutmeg, and salt.

3. Add the ghee and mix thoroughly.

4. While the paste is still warm and runny, pour it into a labeled glass container. Let it cool, then cover and refrigerate. The mixture will thicken as it cools. It may be stored in the refrigerator for up to 3 weeks.

To make the golden milk

5. In a small saucepan, gently heat the milk over low heat until it's warm but not hot.

6. Add 1 or 2 teaspoons of the turmeric paste to the warmed milk.

7. Add your desired sweetener.

Breathe Easy Syrup

This simple syrup can help break up congestion and open up the breathing passages. When you feel an asthmatic episode coming on, take 1 teaspoon of this syrup.

**MAKES 1 CUP
(48 TEASPOON SERVINGS)**

½ **cup raw honey**
½ **cup freshly squeezed
   lemon juice**
1 **(1-inch) piece fresh
   ginger, peeled**
6 **garlic cloves, peeled**
¼ **teaspoon
   cayenne pepper**

1. Put the honey, lemon juice, ginger, garlic, and cayenne in a blender or food processor and puree. Pour into a mason jar or other glass jar, label, and date.

2. Store at room temperature for up to 2 days or in the refrigerator for up to 1 week.

Garlic-Tea Tree Foot Balm

Both garlic and tea tree essential oil are renowned for their ability to combat athlete's foot. However, no essential oil is safe to use undiluted.

**MAKES 6 DOSES (3 DOSES
PER FOOT)**

6 **garlic cloves, peeled**
¼ **teaspoon tea tree
   essential oil, plus
   10 drops**

1. Pulverize the garlic in either a food processor or blender. Transfer the garlic to a small wide-mouthed jar with a lid and add the essential oil and vinegar. Mix thoroughly.

CONTINUED »

¼ **cup apple cider
vinegar, plus
2 tablespoons**

2. Apply up to 2 tablespoons of the resulting paste to the affected areas on each foot, using your hands or a cotton pad. Put on a thick pair of socks and elevate your feet for 15 to 30 minutes. Wash your feet well afterward, dry your feet, and apply a few extra drops of tea tree essential oil diluted in vinegar (10 drops essential oil in 2 tablespoons of vinegar) before putting on clean socks.

3. Repeat once a day for up to 1 week. The vinegar acts as a preservative.

4. Store the remaining balm in a cool, dark place for several weeks.

SAFETY TIP: At one time, it was considered safe to use tea tree, lavender, or patchouli essential oils "neat," or undiluted. This is no longer the case, as it has been found that they can gradually sensitize people, resulting in serious respiratory and allergic reactions that are lifelong. *No* essential oils are safe to use undiluted.

ATHLETE'S FOOT

Tea Tree Foot Powder

This one-two punch of baking soda and tea tree oil combines astringents and anti-fungals to keep feet dry while stopping foot fungus and preventing it from recurring. Use this powder alongside other treatments to maximize its effectiveness.

MAKES 1 CUP

**1 cup baking soda
20 drops tea tree
essential oil**

1. In a medium bowl, combine the baking soda and 5 drops of tea tree essential oil. Blend using a whisk or fork.

2. Add 5 more drops of tea tree essential oil and mix until well blended.

CONTINUED »

3. Repeat step 2 until all 20 drops of essential oil have been mixed in.

4. Using a funnel, transfer the foot powder to a labeled sugar shaker.

5. Apply a liberal amount to your socks and shoes before wearing them, and sprinkle on your feet and between your toes after showering.

6. Use once or twice daily. Store in a cool, dry place.

BACK PAIN

First Chakra Oil Blends

According to Ayurveda teachings, the first chakra (the root chakra or muladhara) is located at the end of the tailbone, and its role focuses on security and survival. Its function is to support healthy skeletal and nervous systems. Both of these oil blends provide the fastest-acting pain relief, compared to most other oils or blends. Essential oils are very concentrated, so it is recommended to dilute them in a carrier oil such as fractionated coconut oil or almond oil. They're also sensitive to heat and light, so be sure to use a dark-colored glass bottle for storing. Many roller bottles are made with thick, anti-shock glass that's resistant to corrosion, and their amber color protects against UV rays. For this recipe, you can use a 10-milliliter roller bottle.

MAKES ⅓ OUNCE

For blend #1

10 mL fractionated coconut oil

1 drop helichrysum essential oil

1 drop myrrh essential oil

2 drops patchouli essential oil

3 drops vetiver essential oil

3 drops ylang-ylang essential oil

CONTINUED »

10 mL fractionated coconut oil

2 drops cypress essential oil

2 drops ylang-ylang essential oil

2 drops eucalyptus essential oil

3 drops ginger essential oil

To make either blend

1. Fill a 10-milliliter dark roller bottle with the fractionated coconut oil. Add the essential oils from either blend and shake to combine.

2. Apply a few drops of this blend to your first chakra. Massage it in to relieve pain. Alternatively, use this blend in a warm compress or diffuser.

BACK PAIN

Ginger, Turmeric, and Cherry Tonic

Ginger and turmeric are a dynamic combination for fighting pain in the body. Turmeric can reduce inflammation, and ginger can stimulate circulation, bringing warmth to the extremities.

MAKES 1 SERVING

1 cup water

1 black tea bag

¼ teaspoon ground ginger

¼ teaspoon ground turmeric

¼ cup tart cherry juice

1. Boil the water.

2. Place the tea bag in a mug. Add the ginger and turmeric.

3. Fill the mug with boiling water.

4. Cover and steep for 3 to 5 minutes.

5. Add the cherry juice to the mug. Remove the tea bag and enjoy.

Calendula-Lavender Blister Balm

Use this simple balm for blisters and other minor injuries to the skin. It is also useful for bug bites, bruises, and burns.

MAKES 4 OUNCES

⅜ cup coconut oil
2 tablespoons
   calendula-infused oil
   (page 30)
20 drops lavender
   essential oil

1. In a double boiler, combine the coconut oil and calendula oil over low heat. Stir until the coconut oil has completely melted.

2. Remove from the heat and let cool for 2 minutes, then stir in the lavender essential oil.

3. Pour into a small jar or tin. Let cool completely, then secure the cap tightly and label the jar.

4. Apply a thin layer of balm to the blister. Top with a bandage or blister pad if needed.

5. Reapply as needed. Keep the balm in a cool, dry place between uses. As long as no moisture is introduced, it will last for up to 1 year.

Chamomile Blister Balm

Chamomile soothes pain while helping blisters heal. This balm is also useful for minor cuts, scrapes, and burns.

MAKES 4 OUNCES

⅜ cup olive oil
2 tablespoons coconut oil
20 drops chamomile
   essential oil

1. In a double boiler, combine the olive oil and coconut oil over low heat. Stir until the coconut oil has completely melted, then remove from the heat and let cool for 2 minutes.

2. Stir in the chamomile essential oil.

CONTINUED »

3. Pour into a small jar or tin. Cool completely, then secure the cap tightly and label the jar.

4. Apply a thin layer of balm to the blister. Top with a bandage or blister pad if needed.

5. Reapply as needed. Keep the balm in a cool, dry place between uses. As long as no moisture is introduced, it will last for up to 1 year.

BRONCHITIS

Smoking Blend for Stubborn Tight Chest Cold

In terms of health, it's generally counterintuitive to smoke anything anymore. But sometimes there may be a therapeutic reason to do so. I've tried a few smoking blends for lung issues and have had great results with this one. Some people use blends to quit smoking. If they work and do no harm, you'll get no judgment from me there. Use freshly dried herbs in this recipe if possible, or dry them yourself.

MAKES ABOUT ¼ CUP

3 tablespoons dried mullein leaf

1 tablespoon dried horehound

1½ teaspoons dried lavender flowers

1 teaspoon dried peppermint

½ teaspoon dried California poppy (optional)

¼ teaspoon dried thyme (optional)

1. Using a coffee grinder, grind the mullein, horehound, lavender, peppermint, California poppy, and thyme (if using) until they are in similar-size bits and are well blended. The mixture should have the consistency of tobacco.

CONTINUED »

2. Use a pipe, rolling papers, or a vaporizer to smoke, taking only one or two inhalations at a time.

3. Store in an airtight container in a cool, dry place, and use within 3 months.

BRONCHITIS

Turmeric Cough Formula

Turmeric eases the inflammation associated with bronchitis, and honey helps soothe coughing and thin secretions. This remedy is safe for children but should not be given to infants less than one year old.

MAKES 1 DOSE

1 cup water
1 teaspoon ground turmeric
1 tablespoon raw honey
1 teaspoon freshly squeezed lemon juice

1. Boil the water and pour it into a mug.

2. Add the turmeric, honey, and lemon juice and stir well. Allow the formula to cool enough to drink.

3. Drink the entire dose on an empty stomach 3 times a day until symptoms subside.

BRUISES

BS Salve

There's no bull here! This salve is soothing and healing, easing the pain of bumps, bruises, and scratches and breaking down the stagnant blood that forms bruises.

CONTINUED »

MAKES ABOUT ½ CUP

2 tablespoons dried
   plantain leaf
2 tablespoons
   dried calendula
1½ tablespoons dried
   lavender flowers
1½ tablespoons dried
   rose petals
1 tablespoon dried basil
1½ cups olive oil
1½ ounces beeswax

1. Follow the instructions in chapter 3 for making an herb-infused oil and a salve (pages 30 and 31) using the dried plantain leaf, calendula, lavender, rose petals, basil, olive oil, and beeswax.

2. Label your salve with the name, ingredient list, and date it was made.

3. Apply liberally as needed to scratches, bumps, and bruises.

4. Store in a cool, dark place for up to 1 year.

BRUISES

Soothing Arnica Salve

This simple arnica salve helps reduce the pain and swelling associated with bruises and is also useful for alleviating the pain associated with arthritis, sore muscles, and minor sprains. Do not apply it to broken skin.

MAKES 20 TO 30 DOSES

½ cup olive oil or
   sunflower oil
2 tablespoons crushed
   dried arnica, or
   4 tablespoons
   fresh arnica
2 tablespoons finely
   grated beeswax

1. Preheat the oven to 200°F.

2. In a medium oven-safe glass or ceramic bowl or baking dish, combine the oil and arnica. Put it in the oven for 3 to 4 hours.

3. After removing the bowl from the oven, allow the mixture to cool.

4. Strain into a separate bowl, extracting as much oil as possible from the arnica. Compost the solids.

5. Combine the oil with the beeswax and heat gently until the beeswax has melted. Mix well and pour into a 4-ounce labeled container.

Aloe Vera–Peppermint Gel

Aloe vera and peppermint combine to take the sting out of bug bites while relieving swelling. Make a batch ahead of time and keep it in the refrigerator indefinitely.

MAKES 8 OUNCES

1 (8-ounce) bottle
alcohol-free aloe
vera gel
20 drops peppermint
essential oil

1. In a large bowl, whisk together the aloe vera gel and peppermint essential oil.

2. Using a funnel, transfer the gel to a labeled plastic squeeze bottle.

3. With your fingertips, apply a small amount to the affected area.

4. Reapply as needed to keep itching and swelling under control.

Cooling Aloe-Lavender Burn Gel

Aloe gel and lavender essential oil are prized for their abilities to soothe and heal burns and reduce the potential for scarring. This easy recipe is a snap to prepare in an emergency.

MAKES 1 TO 5 DOSES

Gel from 1 medium-size
aloe leaf, or
1 tablespoon
commercially prepared
alcohol-free aloe
vera gel

10 drops lavender
essential oil

1. In a small bowl, combine the aloe gel and lavender essential oil, stirring well to ensure that the mixture is completely blended.

CONTINUED »

2. Apply the gel liberally to the affected area, and allow it to evaporate naturally.

3. Reapply as needed, storing the gel in an airtight, labeled container in the refrigerator for up to 3 days.

BURNS, SPLINTERS, BLEMISHES

Plantain Salve

Keep this salve handy for all kinds of household issues. You can put it on burns (after the skin has thoroughly cooled), splinters, blemishes, or anywhere a drawing salve is needed. It should have a noticeable effect pretty quickly. If it doesn't, switch to a poultice without oil.

MAKES SLIGHTLY MORE THAN 4 OUNCES

½ **cup plantain-infused olive oil (page 30)**
½ **ounce beeswax**

1. Heat the oil and beeswax gently in a double boiler until the wax has completely melted and combined with the oil.

2. Pour the salve into small, labeled jars. It will keep for 6 months at room temperature or for 1 year in the refrigerator. You'll know it's no longer good if the oil smells "off."

CANKER SORES

Lemon Balm–Licorice Infusion

Lemon balm and licorice are effective agents against the virus that causes cold sores. If fresh lemon balm is not available, use freeze-dried lemon balm instead.

CONTINUED »

MAKES 1 CUP

1 tablespoon chopped
   fresh lemon
   balm leaves
1 teaspoon dried
   chopped (cut and
   sifted) licorice root
1¼ cups water

1. In a small saucepan, combine the lemon balm and licorice root with the water. Bring the mixture to a boil over medium-high heat, then reduce the heat to low and simmer for 10 minutes.

2. Strain into a mug, using the back of a spoon to press the liquid from the herbs before composting them.

3. Drink hot or iced.

4. Enjoy this infusion 3 to 4 times daily as soon as you notice the tingling that precedes a cold sore.

CANKER SORES

Sage Gargle

Sage is a simple remedy for soothing the sting of canker sores. This gargle is also useful for alleviating the pain and itching associated with coughing and sore throats.

MAKES 16 TO 32 DOSES

2 cups water
3 teaspoons crushed
   dried sage, or
6 teaspoons chopped
   fresh sage leaves

1. In a medium saucepan, combine the water and sage and bring the mixture to a boil over medium heat. Cover the pan with a lid and reduce the heat to low; allow the mixture to simmer for 15 minutes.

2. Remove the saucepan from the heat. Allow the mixture to cool with the lid on the pan to prevent the steam from escaping.

3. Strain into a medium bowl and compost the solids. Pour the liquid into a labeled jar and cover with a tight-fitting lid. Refrigerate, but use within 1 week.

4. Rinse or gargle with 1 to 2 tablespoons of the mixture 3 times a day until symptoms subside.

Hibiscus Tea

Hibiscus is widely consumed around the world and has been used by traditional herbal practitioners to treat high blood pressure. Recent studies show that hibiscus tea can lower blood pressure as effectively as some conventional hypertension drugs. It can open the arteries, slow the release of hormones that constrict blood vessels, and boost immune function. Hibiscus also provides valuable antioxidants and serves as a diuretic.

MAKES 1 SERVING

1 teaspoon dried
   hibiscus flowers
1 cup boiling water

Place the hibiscus into a mug full of boiling water. Steep for 5 minutes, then strain and compost the solids. Drink 3 to 4 cups per day.

CIRCULATION ISSUES

Cold Hands, Warm Heart Tea Blend

Not only does this tea have warming and relaxing properties, but also it's beneficial for your heart and circulatory system.

MAKES 15 (1-CUP) SERVINGS

¼ cup fresh hawthorn
   berries, leaves,
   and twigs
¼ cup fresh
   ginkgo leaves

¼ cup fresh chamomile
   flowers
2 tablespoons fresh
   thyme leaves
2 tablespoons finely
   chopped fresh ginger

Raw honey, for
   sweetening (optional)
Lemon, for serving
   (optional)

CONTINUED »

1. In a large bowl, combine the hawthorn, ginkgo, chamomile, thyme, and ginger.

2. Transfer the tea blend to an airtight container. Label and date the blend.

3. To use, put 1 rounded teaspoon in an infuser and place it in a 10-ounce mug. Cover with boiling water and let steep for 5 to 7 minutes. Remove the infuser. Compost the solids. Sweeten with honey and lemon (if using).

4. Wrap your hands around the warm mug and enjoy up to 3 times a day.

5. Store the loose tea in a cool, dry place out of direct sunlight for up to 1 year.

COLD

Echinacea Cold Care Tea

Echinacea, hyssop, peppermint, and thyme come together to soothe your cold's symptoms and shorten its duration. Make a big batch of the tea blend and keep it on hand so you can begin fighting symptoms as soon as they pop up. Omit the hyssop if you are pregnant.

MAKES 35 DOSES

2 ounces dried chopped (cut and sifted) echinacea root
1 ounce dried hyssop
1 ounce dried peppermint
1 ounce dried thyme

2 cups boiling water (per dose)

Raw honey or stevia, for sweetening (optional)

1. In a medium bowl, combine the echinacea root, hyssop, peppermint, and thyme.

2. Transfer the tea blend to an airtight container. Label and date the blend.

CONTINUED »

3. To prepare a serving of tea, put 2 tablespoons of the dried herb mixture into 2 cups of boiling water and allow the herbs to steep for 10 to 15 minutes.

4. Strain into a large mug. Compost the solids. Sweeten with honey (if using).

5. Drink the entire dose 3 times a day until symptoms subside.

6. Store the loose tea in a cool, dry place out of direct sunlight for up to 1 year.

COLD

Nasturtium Pesto

How's this for delicious medicine? My favorite way to incorporate healing herbs is by adding them to scrumptious meals. Make this pesto ahead and freeze into ¼-cup portions to be used as part of a yummy campaign to prevent illness. Some people don't add the cheese before freezing and instead add it at the time of serving, but I've never had a problem. We use up this pesto pretty quickly in my house.

MAKES ABOUT 3 CUPS

2 cups fresh
   nasturtium leaves
½ cup shelled walnuts
6 garlic cloves, peeled
½ cup freshly grated
   Parmesan cheese
¾ cup olive oil
Hot sauce, for
   seasoning (optional)

1. In a large saucepan, blanch the nasturtium leaves in boiling water for 10 to 15 seconds. Drain and plunge the leaves into ice water to cool. Dry gently on tea towels.

2. Place the leaves, walnuts, garlic, cheese, and olive oil in a blender and blend until smooth. If desired, add a few drops of hot sauce and blend quickly to combine.

3. Drizzle the pesto over pasta or the dish of your choice. Freeze in ¼-cup servings in labeled, airtight resealable bags and use as desired within 3 to 4 months.

Eucalyptus Rub

Eucalyptus vapors help thin mucus, making it easier to expel. There are a few ways to use this aromatic herb—add a few drops of essential oil to a hot bath, tie two or three sprigs under the showerhead, or try this simple rub to ease congestion.

MAKES 16 DOSES

4 tablespoons olive oil
1 teaspoon finely grated beeswax
40 drops eucalyptus essential oil
4 drops peppermint essential oil

1. In a medium saucepan, combine the olive oil and beeswax over low to medium-low heat, stirring just until the beeswax melts into the olive oil.

2. Remove the mixture from the heat, add the eucalyptus and peppermint oils, and stir again.

3. Pour the mixture into a small jar or tin and allow it to cool completely before topping the jar with a tight-fitting lid. Label and date the jar.

4. Rub about 1 teaspoon on your chest as needed.

5. The rub will keep for up to 1 year.

Simmering Potpourri

This potpourri combats viruses, relieves congestion and stuffy nose, and is especially useful in the winter when the air is drier. The steam, combined with the aromatic, cleansing, and health-boosting properties of these herbs, makes this more than an air freshener. This is an all-natural, gentle remedy, and it smells amazing!

CONTINUED »

MAKES 6 TO 7 SIMMERS (EACH CAN BE USED AT LEAST TWICE)

½ cup dried rosemary

½ cup dried eucalyptus leaves

½ cup dried lavender buds

¼ cup dried orange or grapefruit zest

2 tablespoons dried ginger pieces

1. In a labeled pint jar, combine the rosemary, eucalyptus, lavender, orange or grapefruit zest, and ginger.

2. To use, fill a small pot with water, then add about ¼ cup of the blend. Bring to a boil quickly, then reduce the heat to low, or place the pot on top of a woodstove to replace some humidity.

3. As you enjoy the steam and fragrance, keep a watch on the water level.

4. Store the unused potpourri mix in the jar at room temperature indefinitely.

COLD AND COUGH

Garlic and Herb Oxymel

The term oxymel *is from the Latin word* oxymeli, *meaning acid and honey. This is a splendid medium that lends itself well to many different herbal uses. Vinegars help extract vitamins and minerals, as well as the other various properties from herbs. The vinegar itself is the preservative, and oxymels can be used alone as medicine, diluted in hot tea or water to ward off or recover from illness, or incorporated into dressings or marinades for meals.*

MAKES 1 QUART

2½ cups apple cider vinegar

1 cup raw honey

Cloves from 1 head garlic, minced

1 tablespoon fresh thyme leaves

1 tablespoon chopped fresh rosemary leaves

1 tablespoon grated fresh ginger

1. In a 1-quart jar, mix together the vinegar and honey until the honey is mostly dissolved.

CONTINUED »

2. Add the garlic, thyme, rosemary, and ginger.

3. Cover the jar with a nonmetallic cap, or lay plastic wrap across the top and then secure the lid. Label and date the jar.

4. Let steep at room temperature for at least 1 week, shaking the jar daily and before using. This oxymel will keep for up to 1 year.

COLD AND COUGH

Hyssop Tea Blend for Coughs and Colds

This is a great tea to drink when you have gobs of wet, runny mucus. Between the hyssop and the yarrow, the tea will help you get more comfortable, and the elderflowers step in to assist the hyssop in warming the body and inducing a sweat. If pregnant, leave the hyssop out of the recipe and increase the peppermint to ½ cup.

MAKES ABOUT 14 TABLESPOONS

½ cup dried hyssop
¼ cup dried elderflower
1 tablespoon
  dried yarrow
1 tablespoon
  dried peppermint
1 tablespoon dried
  ginger pieces
1 cup boiling water

Raw honey, for
  sweetening (optional)

Freshly squeezed
lemon juice, for
  serving (optional)

1. In a medium bowl, mix together the hyssop, elder-flowers, yarrow, peppermint, and ginger.

2. Place a heaping tablespoon of the blend into a tea ball, and lower it into the boiling water.

3. Cover and steep for 5 to 10 minutes. Compost the solids.

CONTINUED »

4. Add honey and lemon juice (if using). The acid of the lemon helps cut through mucus during a wet cold, so use plenty.

5. Refrigerate in a jar for up to 4 days. Drink as needed.

COLD AND COUGH

Triple Ginger Elixir

This is a delicious drink to sip after dinner, and it also packs a powerful medicinal punch—you can take it by the tablespoonful when you're sick. When you add a spoonful to hot tea, you can reap all the incredible benefits of ginger by the mugful. The ingredients are very flexible, so if you can't find one or two of them, don't let that stop you. As long as you have ginger, honey, and lemon, you're good to go.

MAKES ABOUT 3 CUPS

½ cup chopped
  fresh ginger
¼ cup chopped
  fresh turmeric
1½ tablespoons dried
  galangal pieces, or
  ¼ cup chopped fresh
1 lemon, thinly sliced
1 tablespoon chopped
  dried cinnamon bark
  (aka cinnamon chips)
2 star anise pods

5 cardamom pods
1 cup raw honey

2 to 3 cups 100-proof
  vodka or brandy

1. In a 1-quart jar, combine the ginger, turmeric, galangal, lemon slices, cinnamon, star anise, cardamom pods, and honey. Pour in enough of the vodka/brandy to completely cover the ingredients.

2. Cover and label the jar and let steep for about a month.

3. Strain, compost the solids, and enjoy. Store in a cool place out of direct sunlight. This elixir can keep for a minimum of 5 years.

Super Elderberry Syrup

Elderberry syrup is very easy to make and can help fight the common cold and flu. The dark purple elderberry is known for having powerful natural antiviral effects that can help lessen the symptoms of a cold and the flu. This recipe also contains clove and raw honey, which contain antioxidants and natural antiviral and antifungal properties. Adults can take 1 tablespoon daily; children can take 1 teaspoon daily.

MAKES ABOUT 3 CUPS

1 cup dried elderberries

4 cups water

1 cinnamon stick

1 (2-inch) piece fresh ginger, peeled

1 teaspoon dried cloves

3 or 4 slices dried chopped (cut and sifted) astragalus root

2 tablespoons dried chopped (cut and sifted) echinacea root

1 cup raw honey

1. In a large pot, combine the elderberries, water, cinnamon stick, ginger, cloves, astragalus root, and echinacea root and bring to a boil over medium heat.

2. Reduce the heat to low and continue to simmer for 45 minutes or until the liquid is reduced by about half.

3. Remove the pot from the heat and allow the liquid to cool completely.

4. Using a piece of cheesecloth or a nut bag, strain the elderberry mixture into a medium bowl.

5. Add the honey and whisk gently to combine. (Make sure the liquid has completely cooled so the heat doesn't kill the beneficial enzymes in the honey.)

6. Transfer to a labeled and dated quart jar and store in the refrigerator for up to 1 year.

Tulsi Rose Tea Blend

This is a bright, flavorful herbal tea that tastes good and is both cheering and antiviral. This is especially powerful for cold and flu prevention. Drink it regularly during the winter months or at the first signs of a cold. I really like to trim, zest, and dry the lemon peel myself, although you can buy dried lemon zest commercially. Everything else comes from the summer garden or the farmers' market.

MAKES ABOUT 30 CUPS

½ cup dried holy basil

¼ cup dried rose petals

2 tablespoons dried
spearmint leaves

2 tablespoons
dried elderberries

1 tablespoon dried
lemon zest

1. In a labeled and dated jar, mix together the basil, rose, spearmint, elderberries, and lemon zest. The elderberries tend to sink to the bottom, so keep that in mind when filling a tea ball.

2. For each cup of tea, put a heaping teaspoon of the blend in a tea ball, place it in a mug, and pour hot water into the mug. Steep for 5 to 10 minutes. You can remove the herbs or let them continue to steep while you drink.

3. Store the loose tea in a cool, dry place out of direct sunlight for up to 1 year.

Yarrow and Chamomile Tea

This is a tea you can make if you have a cold or flu accompanied by a fever. Yarrow is thought to have both anti-inflammatory and antimicrobial properties. In ancient times, it was called herbe militaris, *or the military herb, because it was often used to halt bleeding and heal wounds. Both yarrow and elderflower are considered diaphoretic, meaning they induce sweating by gently raising body temperature. Chamomile is a classic herb that promotes*

CONTINUED »

relaxation and deep sleep. Yarrow does have a slightly bitter taste, which can be masked by adding raw honey and lemon—both of which have the added benefit of being natural cough suppressants.

MAKES 1 SERVING

1 teaspoon dried yarrow

1 teaspoon dried
   chamomile flowers

1 teaspoon dried
   elderflower (optional)

3 or 4 fresh peppermint
   leaves (optional)

1 cup hot water

1 teaspoon raw honey

Squeeze of fresh lemon
   juice (optional)

1. Place the yarrow and chamomile in a French press. (Include the elderflower and peppermint if using.)

2. Pour the hot water into the French press.

3. Cover and let steep for 30 minutes, then press the plunger down and pour the tea into a mug. Compost the solids.

4. Sweeten with honey, add the lemon juice (if using), and enjoy.

CONSTIPATION

Ginger-Fennel Infusion

Ginger and fennel increase blood flow to the intestinal tract and gently alleviate constipation. This remedy may ease other gastrointestinal symptoms, too, like gas, cramps, or bloating.

MAKES 1 CUP

2 tablespoons grated
   fresh ginger

1 tablespoon
   fennel seeds

1 tablespoon raw honey

1¼ cups water

1. In a small saucepan, combine the ginger, fennel, honey, and water and bring them to a boil over medium-high heat.

2. Reduce the heat to medium-low and simmer the herbs for 15 minutes.

CONTINUED »

3. Strain into a mug, using the back of a spoon to press the liquid from the herbs before composting them.

4. Drink 2 to 3 cups daily while constipated.

Cinnamon-Chamomile Cough Syrup

This natural cough syrup soothes sore throats, eases coughing, and helps you rest. It is safe for children but should not be given to infants under one year old.

MAKES 32 ADULT DOSES OR 96 CHILD DOSES (3 CUPS)

4 cups water
¼ cup grated fresh ginger
¼ cup dried chamomile flowers, or ½ cup fresh chamomile flowers
1 tablespoon ground cinnamon
1 cup raw honey

1. In a medium saucepan, combine the water, ginger, chamomile, and cinnamon and bring the mixture to a boil over medium-high heat. Reduce the heat to medium-low and allow the mixture to simmer gently for 15 to 20 minutes, until its volume has reduced by half.

2. Remove the saucepan from the heat and allow the mixture to cool until it is safe to handle, then strain into a medium bowl and compost the solids. Pour the strained liquid back into the saucepan and add the honey, heating gently to combine thoroughly.

3. Pour the syrup into a jar and allow it to cool completely before capping it with a tight-fitting lid. Label and date the jar.

4. Adults can take 1 tablespoon, 3 to 5 times a day. Children over the age of 1 year can take 1 teaspoon, 3 to 5 times a day.

5. Store the cough syrup in the refrigerator for up to 1 month.

Cough Calmer Syrup

Coughs come in many forms, including a tickling cough; a dry, unproductive cough; and a wet, barking cough. They can also be hot and painful or more on the cold side. This syrup helps clear excess mucus from the lungs, soothing spasmodic coughs.

MAKES 3 CUPS

4 cups water

2 tablespoons dried basil

2 tablespoons dried raspberry leaf

2 tablespoons dried peppermint

1 tablespoon dried peach leaf

1 tablespoon dried mullein leaves

½ red onion, chopped

1 cup raw honey

1. In a medium saucepan, combine the water, basil, raspberry leaf, peppermint, peach leaf, mullein, and onion; bring the mixture to a boil over medium-high heat. Reduce the heat to medium-low and allow the mixture to simmer gently for 15 to 20 minutes, until its volume has reduced by half.

2. Remove the saucepan from the heat and allow the mixture to cool until it is safe to handle, then strain into a medium bowl and compost the solids. Pour the strained liquid back into the saucepan and add the honey, heating gently to combine thoroughly.

3. Pour the syrup into a jar and allow it to cool completely before capping it with a tight-fitting lid. Label and date the jar.

4. Adults can take 1 to 3 teaspoons as needed. Halve this dose for children under 12.

5. Store the cough syrup in the refrigerator for up to 1 month.

Rose 'n' Herb Cough Syrup

This syrup is yummy and effective. All the herbs work together to moisten, tone, and soothe the throat and upper-respiratory system. Even the little ones in the house will happily take this syrup, but it should not be given to infants less than one year old.

MAKES ABOUT 1 QUART

2 cups dried rose petals
½ cup dried peppermint
¼ cup dried plantain leaf
2 tablespoons
   dried sage
2 tablespoons dried
   mullein flowers
4 cups water
1½ cups sugar
½ cup raw honey

1. Combine the rose petals, peppermint, plantain, sage, mullein flowers, and water in a food processor and process to form a very thin slush.

2. Transfer the mixture to a 2-quart saucepan. Cover the pan and bring the mixture to a boil over high heat. Reduce the heat to low and simmer for 15 minutes.

3. Remove from the heat. Strain the liquid well and compost the solids.

4. Return the liquid to the pan and bring it to a boil over high heat.

5. Add the sugar and stir until it is completely dissolved. Continue to boil for 3 to 5 minutes, until the mixture has begun to thicken.

6. Stir in the honey.

7. Remove from the heat and let the cough syrup cool slightly before pouring it into labeled, dated bottles.

8. Adults can take 1 tablespoon, 3 to 5 times a day. Children over the age of 1 year can take 1 teaspoon, 3 to 5 times a day.

9. Store the syrup in the refrigerator for up to 1 year.

Thyme and Elderberry Cough Drops

You can make these terrific cough soothers with any herb that calms coughs and scratchy throats.

MAKES 100 TO 300 DROPS, DEPENDING ON SIZE OF THE CANDY

1½ cups water
2 tablespoons
  dried elderberries
1 tablespoon
  dried thyme
3 cups granulated sugar
2 tablespoons butter,
  plus more for greasing
Confectioners' sugar,
  for coating

1. In a medium saucepan, start the thyme and elderberry infusion by bringing the water to a boil over high heat. Add the elderberries and thyme, reduce the heat to medium-low, and simmer for 15 minutes.

2. Remove the pan from the heat, cover, and let steep for 1 hour. If you have less than 1 cup of liquid, add water until you have 1 cup. If you have more than 1 cup, simmer a bit more until you have 1 cup. Strain into a 1-cup glass measuring cup. Set aside.

3. Coat a large glass baking dish with butter. Set aside.

4. In a large, heavy saucepan off the heat, combine the thyme-elderberry infusion, granulated sugar, and butter, stirring to dissolve the sugar. Turn the heat to medium-high. If cooked too fast, the mixture will try to climb out of the pan and scorch. Boil the mixture until it reaches 300°F on a candy thermometer.

5. Remove the pan from the heat and stir for a minute, then pour the mixture into the prepared baking dish.

6. Sprinkle a clean work surface or baking sheet with confectioners' sugar.

CONTINUED »

7. As the mixture cools, pull up the end of the candy with a fork. Using kitchen shears, cut the candy into pieces and toss in the confectioners' sugar, where it will finish hardening. You can put it in a warm oven (180°F to 200°F, "warm" setting) if the candy is setting up too fast. When the candy sets up, it is hard.

8. Store the cough drops in a labeled, dated jar in a cool, dry place for up to 1 year.

CROHN'S DISEASE

Gut-Loving Piña Colada Kefir

This delicious gut-soothing probiotic drink is sweet and tangy with a little fizz. Water kefir is a naturally fermented drink packed with living probiotics and enzymes, and additional probiotics are present in the coconut water and vinegar.

MAKES 4 SERVINGS

2 to 4 tablespoons coconut water kefir

½ cup fresh aloe vera gel

½ cup pineapple juice

Juice of 1 lemon

½ teaspoon ground ginger

2 teaspoons apple cider vinegar

½ cup water

1. Combine the coconut water kefir, aloe vera, pineapple juice, lemon juice, ginger, vinegar, and water in a labeled, dated glass jar. Shake well.

2. This concoction can be stored in the refrigerator for up to 3 days. Drink ½ cup each day for maximum benefits.

Calendula First-Aid Salve

Calendula is a natural antibiotic, and it speeds healing by promoting tissue regeneration. Make this natural first-aid salve ahead of time for use anytime you suffer from a minor cut or scrape.

MAKES 100 DOSES

1 cup olive oil or
   sunflower oil
½ cup crushed dried
   calendula flowers,
   or 1 cup fresh
   calendula flowers
4 tablespoons finely
   grated beeswax

1. Preheat the oven to 200°F.

2. In a glass or ceramic oven-safe bowl or baking dish, combine the oil and calendula and put it in the oven, uncovered, for 3 to 4 hours.

3. After removing the mixture from the oven, allow it to cool. Strain the mixture, extracting as much oil as possible from the calendula. Compost the solids.

4. Pour the oil back into the oven-safe container and add the beeswax. Put the container back in the oven and leave it there for a few minutes, or until the beeswax has melted.

5. After removing it from the oven, stir the salve well to blend it. Carefully transfer it to a labeled and dated jar or tin. Allow the salve to cool completely before capping.

6. Apply the salve on the affected area as needed. Store in a cool, dark place for no more than 6 months.

Cuts and Scrapes Dusting Powder

This powder helps with clotting, keeping germs at bay, reducing pain, and healing wounds. Because it is a powder, versus a salve or oil, it helps dry out especially weepy wounds.

MAKES ABOUT 20 APPLICATIONS

2 teaspoons echinacea
   root powder

1 teaspoon marshmallow
   root powder

1 teaspoon ground
   lavender

1 teaspoon comfrey
   root powder

1 teaspoon
   calendula powder

1. In a small bowl, mix together the echinacea, marshmallow root, lavender, comfrey root, and calendula until well combined.

2. Pour the powder mixture into a jar with a shaker top (an empty spice jar that's been washed works great), and label with the ingredients and instructions for use.

3. Shake the powder onto a cleaned wound to fill it. If needed, cover with a bandage to hold the powder in place. Apply 2 to 3 times a day or as needed if the wound is weeping. Store in a cool, dry, dark place (out of direct sunlight), where it should retain usefulness for at least 1 year.

Lavender Baby Balm

Coconut oil creates a soothing barrier that prevents moisture and naturally occurring compounds found in urine and feces from causing a baby's diaper rash to worsen, while lavender essential oil helps keep bacteria at bay. If your baby has a fever, diarrhea, or areas of infection associated with the diaper rash, see your pediatrician immediately.

CONTINUED »

MAKES 10 DOSES

¼ cup coconut oil
2 teaspoons
  cocoa butter
15 drops lavender
  essential oil

1. In a small pan over low heat, melt the coconut oil and cocoa butter. When they are liquid, remove from the heat and add the lavender oil, mixing well.

2. Pour the mixture into a wide-mouth container, allow it to cool, and put the lid on tightly. Label and date the container, store it in a cool, dry place, and use it within 6 months.

3. Apply a generous coat of the balm after each diaper change. Be sure to change soiled diapers immediately, both to speed healing and to prevent diaper rash in the future.

DIGESTIVE ISSUES

Cinnamon Honey

All the medicinal properties of cinnamon are at your fingertips with this delicious and versatile honey "medicine." Spread it on buttered toast, add it to green tea, toss a spoonful into a meat dish, or just eat it by the spoonful. The honey complements the cinnamon and has lots of health benefits on its own.

MAKES 12 OUNCES

1 cup raw honey
½ cup ground
  (fresh, if possible)
  Ceylon cinnamon

1. Pour the honey into a small bowl. If it seems too thick, you can heat it a little bit: Simply place the container of honey in a bowl of hot water, or in the microwave in 30-second increments, until it thins.

2. Carefully add the cinnamon a little at a time, stirring well.

3. Spoon the flavored honey into a labeled jar or two. Store the jar(s) in a cool, dry place for up to 1 year.

Dandelion Chai Mix

All the spices in this delicious chai are immune stimulating and antibiotic, and many are antiviral and anti-inflammatory. Mixed together, they make for a spicy, sweet, comforting treat.

MAKES 40 (1-CUP) SERVINGS

1 cup chopped fresh
dandelion root,
cut into small,
uniform pieces
2 tablespoons
whole peppercorns
3 tablespoons
cardamom pods
3 tablespoons chopped
dried cinnamon bark
(aka cinnamon chips)
¼ cup dried
ginger pieces
1 cup black tea leaves
(or use rooibos if you
prefer decaf)
½ cup dried dandelion
leaves, crumbled
2 vanilla beans, cut into
small pieces
1 to 1¼ cups water
Raw honey, for
sweetening
Light cream or half-and-
half, for serving

1. Preheat the oven to 200°F.

2. Arrange the dandelion root pieces in a single layer on a baking sheet. Roast for 30 minutes or until they turn dark brown and are completely dried.

3. In a mini food processor or coffee grinder, process the peppercorns, cardamom pods, cinnamon chips, and ginger pieces until you have small, uniform bits. Mix in the black tea, dandelion leaves and roots, and vanilla beans until well combined. Transfer to a labeled, dated glass jar and secure the lid.

4. To use, put 1 rounded teaspoon in an infuser or muslin bag. In a small saucepan, bring the water to a boil over high heat. Place the tea infuser in the pan, cover, and let steep for 15 to 20 minutes. Remove the infuser and compost the solids. Serve the tea in mugs with honey and light cream.

5. Store the loose chai in a cool, dry place out of direct sunlight for up to 1 year.

Dandelion Vinegar

Apple cider vinegar is becoming more and more popular, with a long list of health benefits on its own before we even add the herbs! Using vinegar is an easy way to add the vitamins and minerals packed into all parts of the dandelion plant into many kinds of dishes. You can also just take a tablespoon of the vinegar mixed in a little water. Use this with oil to dress a salad, spritz on cooked veggies, or deglaze a pan and make a light sauce for meat.

MAKES 3½ CUPS

1 cup chopped fresh
　dandelion roots
1 cup fresh dandelion
　leaves, torn into
　small pieces
1 cup fresh
　dandelion flowers
1 quart apple
　cider vinegar

1. Put the dandelion roots, leaves, and flowers in a large, labeled jar and cover with the apple cider vinegar.

2. Line the lid with plastic wrap or wax paper (vinegar will corrode a metal top) and let steep in a cool, dry place for 4 to 6 weeks.

3. When the steeping is done, strain the vinegar, compost the solids, and use in any dish you desire. Store in a cool, dry place out of direct sunlight for 12 to 18 months.

Digestivi-Tea Blend

This tea is tasty and eases many symptoms of poor digestion, such as cramps, bloating, indigestion, and nausea. Some people have trouble swallowing when they're really struggling emotionally. A little liquid can help get the action started, but it's even better to drink a nice hot tea with herbs specifically blended for nervous digestion.

CONTINUED »

MAKES 15 (1-CUP) SERVINGS

¼ **cup dried catnip**
¼ **cup chopped**
  fresh ginger
¼ **cup dried lemon balm**

1. In a large bowl, combine the catnip, ginger, and lemon balm.

2. Transfer the tea blend to an airtight container. Label and date the blend.

3. To use, put 1 rounded teaspoon in an infuser and place it in a 10-ounce mug. Cover with boiling water and let steep for 5 to 7 minutes. Remove the infuser. Compost the solids. This is particularly good after meals. Drink up to 3 times a day.

4. Store the loose tea in a cool, dry place out of direct sunlight for up to 1 year.

DIGESTIVE ISSUES

Fennel Digestive Pastilles

These pastilles are great for assisting with the relief of gas, bloating, stomach upsets, and other digestive complaints. Store a small bottle in your purse or bag for on-the-go relief.

MAKES 10 PASTILLES

1 **tablespoon ground**
  fennel seeds, plus
  more for dusting
2 **teaspoons raw honey**

1. Put the ground fennel seeds in a small bowl, then drizzle the honey over them, stirring to combine as you drizzle. If the mixture forms a stiff paste before you finish, stop drizzling the honey. If it's still sticky and soft, add more powder.

2. Put some extra fennel powder in a separate small bowl. Coat your hands with fennel powder.

3. Pinch off a small piece of the dough, about the size of a pea, and roll it into a ball.

CONTINUED »

4. Roll the ball in the fennel powder, then put it in a labeled, dated glass jar. Repeat until all the pastilles have been formed.

5. Eat 1 pastille 15 to 20 minutes before a meal for improved digestion. For indigestion, gas, and bloating, take 1 or 2 as needed.

6. Store the jar in a cool, dry place for up to 1 year.

DIGESTIVE ISSUES

Homemade Hot Sauce

Adding hot and spicy capsicum to meals is a good way to reap the medicinal benefits of peppers. Having a bottle of this hot sauce on hand makes it easy to season and spice up your meals. It packs a big punch in both flavor and healing. Word to the wise: Wear gloves while preparing this, since it is very hard to get all the oil off your hands.

MAKES ABOUT 2 CUPS

1½ cups rice vinegar
2 dozen small to
  medium red chiles
  (I like a mixture of
  whatever is available),
  coarsely chopped
½ medium red
  bell pepper,
  coarsely chopped
1 medium onion, diced
5 garlic cloves, chopped
½ teaspoon salt

1. In a medium saucepan, combine the vinegar, chiles, bell pepper, onion, garlic, and salt and bring to a boil over medium-high heat.

2. Reduce the heat to medium-low and simmer for about 10 minutes, until the peppers are soft.

3. Using an immersion blender, puree the mixture into a liquid.

4. Simmer, uncovered, for about 5 minutes, until the sauce has reduced slightly.

5. Pour the hot sauce into labeled and dated bottles. Store in the refrigerator for up to 3 months.

Nervous Tummy Tincture

In our family, we call it "feeling urp-y." You know, when there's too much acid and gas, and everything either sits in the gut for a long time (making you feel miserable) or flies through your intestines (resulting in flatulence). Turn to this handy tincture when you need to calm and soothe your digestive tract.

MAKES 4 OUNCES

3 tablespoons
  thyme tincture
3 tablespoons
  chamomile tincture
2 tablespoons
  spearmint tincture

1. In a measuring cup, combine the thyme, chamomile, and spearmint tinctures.

2. Transfer the mixture into a 4-ounce dropper bottle.

3. Label and date the tincture blend.

4. Take 1 to 2 dropperfuls (25 to 50 drops) added to herbal, green, or weak black tea 2 to 3 times a day.

5. Store the tincture blend in a cool, dark place, where it will last for several years.

Yarrow and Chamomile Bitters

Bitter tastes have all but disappeared from most of our diets, but we need them for proper digestion. Bitterness signals to the entire digestive tract that food is coming. It immediately triggers salivation, and all along the digestive route, preparations are made to efficiently process the fuel and move it out.

MAKES 8 TO 10 OUNCES

¼ cup dried yarrow
¼ cup dried
  chamomile flowers

2 tablespoons
  fennel seeds
2 tablespoons
  cardamom pods

2 tablespoons dried
  chopped (cut and
  sifted) licorice root
1¼ cups
  100-proof vodka

CONTINUED »

1. Combine the yarrow, chamomile, fennel seeds, cardamom pods, and licorice root in a mortar and pestle or coffee grinder, and crush but do not powder them. Just break them to release their flavors.

2. Transfer the mixture to a 1-pint jar and cover with the vodka. Seal the jar, label and date it, and let steep for 1 month.

3. Strain, compost the solids, and use by the scant dropper (10 to 20 drops) before meals to promote healthy digestion. This can be stored in a cool, dry place out of direct sunlight for up to 5 years.

EARACHE

Soothing Garlic Ear Drops

Thanks to its antibacterial and antifungal properties, fresh garlic is an excellent herb for treating earaches. When combined with "sweet oil," which is purified olive oil that is normally available at pharmacies and other retailers, garlic soothes pain and promotes healing. This oil can be used by the drop as a flavoring in cooking, too. Sweet almond oil can be substituted if you can't find sweet oil.

MAKES 100 DOSES

⅛ **cup sweet oil**
2 garlic cloves, crushed

1. In a small saucepan, combine the sweet oil and garlic and heat the oil over low heat for 30 minutes, checking frequently to be sure that the oil is only warm, not hot—you don't want the garlic to cook.

2. Strain the oil, compost the garlic, and allow the oil to cool to body temperature. Pour strained oil into a 1-ounce dropper bottle and store in the

CONTINUED »

refrigerator between uses for up to 1 year, warming it to body temperature before each treatment.

3. To use, lie down on your side with the affected ear facing up. Use an eyedropper to place 5 to 7 drops of oil in the ear. Place a cotton ball into the ear for 10 to 15 minutes to keep the oil in place, then allow the remaining oil to evaporate naturally. Repeat 4 times a day for up to 3 days.

EYE ITCH

Itchy Eye Relief Eye Wash

Allergies, sties, and conjunctivitis can make eyes dry, irritated, and itchy. Use this eye wash formula to help soothe them and encourage healing.

MAKES 4 (1-CUP) TREATMENTS

2 teaspoons
   dried elderflower
2 teaspoons dried
   chamomile flowers
2 teaspoons dried basil
2 teaspoons
   dried thyme
1 cup boiling water
1 teaspoon sea salt
   per dose

1. In a small bowl, combine the elderflower, chamomile, basil, and thyme. Transfer to an airtight container and label with the date, ingredients, and directions that follow.

2. Steep 2 teaspoons of tea blend in the boiling water for 15 to 20 minutes. Add 1 teaspoon of sea salt to the tea as it steeps, stirring to dissolve. Once cooled, strain and compost the solids.

3. Pour the liquid into an eye cup. Lean forward, placing the eye cup tightly against your eye with your eye open. Sit or stand upright, flip your head back, blink several times, then lean forward again.

4. Rinse the cup with hot, soapy water, then repeat with the other eye, even if it's not affected. Repeat 4 to 5 times daily until the eyes are completely clear of any irritation.

Willow Bark Decoction

Willow bark is an effective treatment for fever, and sweet herbs such as cinnamon and ginger help mellow its bitter taste. This remedy is also excellent for pain relief, including sore throat and body aches associated with the flu. It is not safe for children.

MAKES 1 DOSE

2 cups water

2 teaspoons chopped
  or crushed dried
  willow bark

1 teaspoon
  ground cinnamon

1 teaspoon
  ground ginger

Raw honey or stevia, for
  sweetening (optional)

1. In a medium saucepan, combine the water, willow bark, cinnamon, and ginger and bring the mixture to a boil over medium-high heat. Reduce the heat to low and allow the mixture to simmer for 20 minutes, uncovered.

2. Strain the liquid into a large mug. Compost the solids.

3. Sweeten with a little honey (if using) before drinking.

4. Drink the entire dose. Repeat up to 4 times per day.

Elderberry Liqueur

With elderberry, medicine doesn't have to taste bad. A small glass of this liqueur sipped each evening during winter will go a long way toward keeping you healthy and happy, and it's a delicious way to unwind after a long day.

MAKES ABOUT 6 CUPS

1 quart fresh
  elderberries

2 cups sugar

Juice and zest
  of 1 lemon

1 (750-mL) bottle
  80-proof vodka

CONTINUED »

1. In a large bowl, using a potato masher or pestle, crush the elderberries and sugar together. Let stand for about 1 hour.

2. Stir in the lemon zest and juice.

3. Transfer the mixture to a clean 2-quart container and add the vodka.

4. Cover, label, date, and let age in a cool, dark place for 1 month.

5. After a month, use a fine-mesh strainer to strain the liqueur. Compost the solids.

6. Transfer the liqueur to decorative glass bottles.

7. You can enjoy this liqueur immediately, but the flavor does continue to develop over time. For the best flavor, age the liqueur for at least another month.

FLU

Elderberry Syrup

In this version of elderberry syrup, the brandy is mostly used as a slight preservative. You can omit it or double it as preferred. This syrup is tasty enough that kids ask for it, and it can be used as a tea sweetener, on pancakes, or on ice cream. It can also be used as a condiment for food, making it a very convenient way to add elder to the family diet. During an illness, take 1 tablespoon of the syrup 4 times a day.

CONTINUED »

MAKES ABOUT 2 QUARTS

2 quarts fresh
  elderberries
2½ pounds sugar
1 cup dried elderflower
1½ teaspoons
  ground cloves
1 tablespoon finely
  chopped dried
  cinnamon bark (aka
  cinnamon chips)
1 cup brandy

1. In a large saucepan over medium heat, cook the elderberries for a few minutes, until they start to burst. Mash the berries with the back of a large spoon to release their juices.

2. Using a mesh strainer or several layers of cheese-cloth, strain the juice and compost the solids. You'll need about 1 quart of juice.

3. Gently wipe out the same saucepan, then return the juice to the pan and add the sugar, elderflower, cloves, and cinnamon chips. Simmer over low heat for 20 minutes.

4. Remove from the heat, let cool, then strain. Compost the solids.

5. Once the syrup has cooled, add the brandy. Pour the finished syrup into bottles or jars, label and date them, and store in the refrigerator for up to 1 year.

FLU

Flu Fighter Tea

When you've got an aching body, wracking headache, fever, chills, and sore throat and just want to sleep but you're too miserable, this tea can help ease the aches and pains and help you sweat out a fever.

MAKES 14 (1-CUP) SERVINGS

¼ cup dried echinacea
  leaves and flowers

¼ cup crushed dried
  rose hips
2 tablespoons
  dried peppermint

2 tablespoons
  dried elderflower

CONTINUED »

1 tablespoon chopped
dried cinnamon bark
(aka cinnamon chips)
1 tablespoon
dried yarrow

1. In a small bowl, combine the echinacea, rose hips, peppermint, elderflower, cinnamon, and yarrow. Transfer to an airtight container and label with the date, ingredients, and instructions for use.

2. To use, put 1 rounded teaspoon of the tea blend in an infuser and lower it into a mug full of boiling water. Let steep for 15 to 20 minutes, then remove the infuser. Compost the solids.

3. Drink 1 cup every couple of hours.

4. Store the loose tea in a cool, dry place out of direct sunlight for up to 1 year.

FLU

Licorice-Echinacea Tea

Echinacea, licorice root, and barberry bark come together to fight flu symptoms in this simple yet effective herbal tea. The barberry bark helps fight diarrhea, the echinacea quells the virus, and the licorice root soothes the digestive tract while coating the throat. This remedy is great for flu and cold alike and is safe for children. Make this dried herb tea in advance and start taking this remedy at the first sign of the flu or a cold to alleviate the symptoms and shorten the duration of the virus. Omit the licorice root in this recipe if you are pregnant or have high blood pressure.

MAKES 15 (½-CUP) DOSES

1 ounce dried chopped
(cut and sifted)
echinacea root

1 ounce dried chopped
(cut and sifted)
licorice root
1 ounce chopped dried
barberry bark

2 cups water per dose
Raw honey or stevia, for
sweetening (optional)

CONTINUED »

1. In a small bowl, mix together the echinacea root, licorice root, and barberry bark. Transfer to a glass container with a lid, label, and date.

2. When symptoms first appear, place the water and 2 teaspoons of the herbal blend in a medium saucepan. Bring the mixture to a boil over medium-high heat. Reduce the heat to low and simmer for 5 minutes.

3. Remove the mixture from the heat, cover it with a lid, and allow it to steep for 15 minutes. Strain the liquid into a mug and compost the solids. Add the honey (if using) and drink.

4. Adults should drink ½ cup of the full-strength tea up to 3 times a day. For children, mix the tea with equal parts of the child's favorite juice. Administer ½ cup at a time up to 3 times a day.

GINGIVITIS

Aloe Mouthwash

Gargling with aloe is terrific for your gums and helps prevent gingivitis. It can also be helpful for sore throats. You can even give it a try the next time you can't wait for that cheese pizza to cool and end up with the roof of your mouth painfully blistered. Aloe juice is made by pressing the entire leaf of the aloe, including the outer green part. It is much easier to work with than aloe gel, which can get sticky. The juice is perfect for this recipe.

CONTINUED »

MAKES 1 CUP

½ cup aloe juice

½ cup water

2 teaspoons
  baking soda

1 drop spearmint
  essential oil

1 drop tea tree
  essential oil

1 drop orange
  essential oil

1. Combine the aloe juice, water, baking soda, spearmint oil, tea tree oil, and orange oil in a 10- or 12-ounce jar, cover, and shake well to dissolve the baking soda.

2. To use, swish an ounce or so of the juice in your mouth for 30 seconds to a minute, then spit it out. Do not swallow.

3. Seal, label, and date the jar and store in the refrigerator. Use within 1 week.

GINGIVITIS

Chamomile Mouth Rinse

Chamomile essential oil is a powerful anti-inflammatory and antiseptic agent. It also serves as a mild analgesic, soothing the discomfort that often accompanies gingivitis.

MAKES 16 TO 32 DOSES

1 cup alcohol-free witch
  hazel hydrosol

1 cup water

6 drops chamomile
  essential oil

6 drops peppermint
  essential oil

1. Combine the witch hazel, water, chamomile oil, and peppermint oil in a glass container with a tight-fitting lid. Label and store it in the refrigerator until it is used up.

2. To use, shake well and swish an ounce or so of the rinse in your mouth for 30 seconds to a minute, then spit out. Do not swallow.

3. Use this rinse every morning and evening after brushing and flossing until symptoms subside.

Cooling Peppermint Compress

Dabbing a little peppermint essential oil on your forehead or the back of your neck can help relieve headaches quickly. If you're all out of essential oil or want to use a milder remedy, give this cooling peppermint compress a try.

MAKES 1 COMPRESS

2 peppermint tea bags
2 cups boiling water
6 ice cubes
1 (4-by-4-inch)
   soft cloth

1. Place the tea bags in a large bowl and add the boiling water. Use a lid or plate to cover the bowl, allowing the tea bags to steep for at least 20 minutes or until cool.

2. Uncover the bowl, remove the tea bags, and squeeze the liquid they contain back into the bowl. Add the ice cubes.

3. To apply the compress, dip the soft cloth into the liquid, wring it out, and place it on your forehead while resting with your eyes closed. Repeat until symptoms subside.

Headache Helper Formula

Headaches are not much fun. This blend of herbs helps soothe a headache fast, letting you get on with your day. Do not give willow internally to children under the age of 18.

MAKES 2 OUNCES

2 tablespoons
   willow tincture

1 tablespoon
   peppermint tincture

1 tablespoon
   basil tincture

CONTINUED »

1. In a 1-cup glass measuring cup, combine the willow tincture, peppermint tincture, and basil tincture and mix well.

2. Using a small metal funnel (if you have one), or a measuring cup with a spout, pour the tincture blend into a 2-ounce dropper bottle.

3. Tighten the dropper lid on the bottle, and label with the name of the formula and the dosage information. This can be stored in a cool, dry place out of direct sunlight for up to 5 years.

4. Add 1 to 2 dropperfuls (25 to 50 drops) of the tincture blend to a small glass of water or juice and drink. Repeat every 20 to 30 minutes for up to 2 hours.

HEARTBURN AND GASTRIC REFLUX

Cooling Chamomile Infusion

Heartburn is sometimes brought on by stress, and it is often a byproduct of indigestion. Chamomile not only relieves stress, but also soothes indigestion. Honey helps soothe the esophageal lining while aiding digestion and promoting healing.

MAKES 1 DOSE

2 tablespoons dried chamomile flowers, or 4 tablespoons fresh chamomile flowers

2 cups water

2 tablespoons raw honey

1. In a medium saucepan, combine the chamomile flowers and water and bring the water to a boil over medium-high heat. Reduce the heat to low and allow the mixture to simmer for 10 to 15 minutes, until the volume has been reduced by about half.

CONTINUED »

2. Remove the saucepan from the heat and pour the mixture through a fine-mesh sieve into a mug, using the back of a spoon to press any remaining liquid from the flowers. Compost the solids.

3. Add the honey, stirring well to ensure it melts into the infusion. Allow the liquid to cool until it is comfortable to sip.

4. Drink this infusion as often as you like to keep heartburn at bay.

HEMORRHOIDS

Witch Hazel Cleansing Pads

Witch hazel helps shrink swollen rectal tissue and provides immediate relief from the itching and burning sensations caused by hemorrhoids.

MAKES 20 CLEANSING PADS

½ **cup alcohol-free witch hazel hydrosol**

1. Stack 20 cotton pads inside a glass, wide-mouth pint jar with a tight-fitting lid, and gently pour the witch hazel into the jar to cover the pads.

2. Use one of these cleansing pads anytime you feel irritation. If symptoms do not improve within 1 week, see your doctor. Do not flush used pads down the toilet, as they may cause blocked pipes.

Healing Adaptogenic Elixir

There is a category of herbs called adaptogens that are commonly used in traditional Chinese medicine and Ayurveda. Adaptogens may help regulate blood sugar by reducing elevated cortisol and blood sugar levels. Helpful adaptogens include ashwagandha, American ginseng, Asian ginseng, cordyceps, holy basil, reishi, rhodiola, and shilajit. This creamy and luscious elixir tastes like hot chocolate—but with added benefits!

MAKES 2 SERVINGS

1½ cups coconut milk

1 tablespoon raw
cacao powder

½ teaspoon
maca powder

1 teaspoon chia seeds

½ teaspoon ground
cinnamon

½ teaspoon reishi
mushroom powder

½ teaspoon
ashwagandha
root powder

½ teaspoon cordyceps
mushroom powder

Pinch Himalayan salt

Liquid stevia, monk fruit
extract, coconut sugar,
or yacon syrup, for
sweetening (optional)

1. In a small saucepan, warm the coconut milk over medium heat. Add the cacao powder, maca, chia seeds, cinnamon, reishi mushroom, ashwagandha root, cordyceps mushroom, and salt.

2. Transfer the mixture to a blender and blend until creamy and frothy.

3. Add 1 or 2 drops of liquid stevia or monk fruit extract or ½ teaspoon of coconut sugar or yacon syrup (if using).

4. Serve chilled or warm—whichever you prefer!

Calming Boswellia Oil

Frankincense essential oil is typically the purest form of boswellia available. When blended with a light carrier oil, it calms itching and soothes stinging almost immediately. This recipe is easy to make in just a few minutes.

MAKES 10 DOSES

2 tablespoons olive oil
15 drops frankincense
   (boswellia)
   essential oil

1. In a small, dark-colored glass bottle, blend the olive oil and boswellia essential oil. Cover and shake well to ensure it is mixed thoroughly. It can then be stored in a cool, dry place out of direct sunlight for up to 1 year.

2. Apply a thin layer to the affected area and allow it to evaporate naturally. Reapply as needed.

Hives Healer Poultice

Hives can be uncomfortable and irritating, especially for children. This poultice helps soothe and reduce hives. Colloidal oatmeal is oatmeal that's been powdered—a blender or coffee grinder will make short work of this.

MAKES 1 POULTICE

1 tablespoon colloidal
   oatmeal powder
1 tablespoon rhassoul,
   bentonite, or
   French clay
1 teaspoon ground
   chamomile

1 teaspoon
   ground lavender
1 teaspoon rose
   petal powder
1 teaspoon gotu
   kola powder

3 tablespoons
   boiling water
1 teaspoon melted
   coconut oil

CONTINUED »

1. In a small bowl, combine the oatmeal, clay, chamomile, lavender, rose, and gotu kola. Stir in the water and coconut oil.

2. Apply the poultice mixture to the hives and let it dry. Climb into a warm bath and soak with a muslin bagful of uncooked oatmeal. Soak the oatmeal in the water, then squeeze the liquid out of the bag onto the hives.

HORMONAL IMBALANCE

Black Nettle Syrup

This recipe is credited to Adrian White of Deer Nation Herbs. Fortifying the nettles with mineral-rich blackstrap molasses is a stroke of genius. I think blackstrap molasses tastes like brown sugar, and I have no trouble taking the syrup straight. If the taste or smell of this syrup is objectionable to you (the mere mention made my mother shudder), mix it with cereal or hot tea, or bake some molasses cookies.

MAKES ABOUT 4 CUPS

3 cups water
1 cup dried nettles
2 cups raw honey
1½ cups blackstrap molasses

1. In a small saucepan over low heat, combine the water and nettles. Gently simmer for 10 to 15 minutes. Cover the pan and remove it from heat. Steep for 2 to 3 hours.

2. Strain the tea, compost the solids, and transfer the liquid to a clean saucepan.

3. Add the honey and bring up to a simmer again over low heat, until the mixture reaches a consistency you like. I usually reduce it by about one-third.

CONTINUED »

4. While the mixture is still hot, add the molasses and stir. Let cool.

5. Transfer the cooled syrup to your desired container, preferably an amber-tinted glass jar. Label and date it.

6. Store the syrup in the refrigerator for up to 1 year.

HORMONAL IMBALANCE

Herb-Infused Energy Balls

This recipe includes lots of adaptogens that can support hormonal health. Energy balls make the perfect snack and are very easy to make. The process of rolling the "dough" can also be very meditative. The basic recipe is versatile; you can experiment with different flavors and spices.

MAKES ABOUT 75 BALLS (1½ TEASPOONS EACH)

1 cup almond butter or
 nut butter of choice
¼ cup tahini
½ cup raw honey
1 teaspoon
 ground cinnamon
¼ cup coconut flakes
¼ cup raw cacao
 powder, maca
 powder, or
 ashwagandha powder

1. In a medium bowl, combine the nut butter and tahini and mix well. Add the honey, cinnamon, and coconut flakes and mix thoroughly, then mix in the cacao powder.

2. Break the dough into 1-inch pieces and roll them into balls with your hands.

3. Place the energy balls in the refrigerator for at least an hour to allow them to firm up before enjoying.

4. Store leftovers in a tightly sealed, labeled, and dated container in the refrigerator. These should be eaten within 1 month.

Steamed Nettles

Steaming nettles briefly, even for a minute, causes the trichomes to break, rendering them stingless. There is something about the flavor of steamed fresh nettles that is deeply nourishing. To me, they taste as if they can make one whole again.

MAKES ABOUT 1 CUP

4 cups fresh stinging
   nettle leaves
½ cup water
1½ teaspoons butter
Salt

1. Using gloves, transfer the nettle leaves to a colander. Rinse them well under cool running water. Drain.

2. In a small saucepan over high heat, bring the water to a boil.

3. Add the nettles, cover, and boil for 1 minute.

4. Drain, then return to the saucepan. Stir in the butter, season with salt, and serve.

Blue Oat Smoothie

This meal-in-a-glass will help support the nerves and the immune system all day long. I like to include blueberries for their anthocyanins, and the holy basil and astragalus boost the adaptogenic power of this blend. You can also add different herbs and spices, such as some ginger, rose, nettles, or a pinch of lavender.

MAKES 2 (1½-CUP) SMOOTHIES

½ cup old-fashioned
   rolled oats
1 cup milk (any kind),
   plus more as needed

½ cup frozen blueberries
2 tablespoons
   raw honey
1 small banana
½ cup ice

1 teaspoon dried
   holy basil
½ teaspoon astragalus
   root powder

CONTINUED »

Put the oats, milk, blueberries, honey, banana, ice, holy basil, and astragalus root in a blender. Cover tightly and pulse to break up the ice cubes. Continue pulsing until smooth. Check consistency and add more milk if necessary. Serve immediately.

IMMUNITY ISSUES

Fire Cider

This cider is based on Rosemary Gladstar's recipe, with a few personal addi-tions. The amounts listed aren't critical, and you can add or delete anything you want. Many people take a shot of this cider every day, particularly when there are a lot of bugs going around. Another way to use it is by mixing it with water or juice. It can also be blended with a little oil for a salad dressing. Vin-egar that is unrefined and unfiltered contains some of the (good) acetic acid/ bacterial culture that turns apple cider into vinegar, which takes the form of a cloudy substance known as the "mother."

MAKES ABOUT 1 QUART

1 quart apple cider vinegar (with the "mother")

5 Thai chiles or other small hot peppers, chopped

1 large red onion, chopped

⅓ cup dried elderberries, or 1 cup fresh elderberries

3 astragalus root slices, chopped

½ cup grated fresh horseradish

Cloves from 1 head garlic, peeled and chopped

¼ cup grated fresh ginger

1 tablespoon ground turmeric, or 3 tablespoons grated fresh turmeric

Juice of 1 lemon

1 cup raw honey

Water or juice, for serving

CONTINUED »

1. Place the vinegar, chiles, onion, elderberries, astragalus, horseradish, garlic, ginger, turmeric, and lemon juice in a half-gallon container and secure with a nonmetallic lid. Label and date the container.

2. Let steep in a warm, dry place for at least 2 weeks.

3. Strain and compost the solids. Mix in the honey.

4. Store in a cool, dark place and use within 1 year.

IMMUNITY ISSUES

Immunitea

Drink this tea one to three times per day when you feel the very beginnings of illness coming on, or when you're heading into a situation that requires your immune system to be in top shape, such as traveling by plane or otherwise sharing space with sick people. Continue drinking for up to two weeks as needed.

MAKES 50 (1-CUP) SERVINGS

1 cup dried echinacea
1 cup dried elder
½ cup dried rose hips
½ cup dried chopped
  (cut and sifted)
  astragalus root
2 teaspoons grated
  fresh ginger
Raw honey and lemon,
  for serving

1. In a mini food processor or coffee grinder, grind the echinacea, elder, rose hips, astragalus root, and ginger to small, similar-size pieces. Transfer to a glass jar with a lid. Label and date the jar.

2. To use, put 1 rounded teaspoon per serving in an infuser. In a small saucepan, bring water to a boil over high heat. Put the infuser in the pan. Reduce the heat to low and simmer for 30 minutes or more. Remove the infuser. Compost the solids.

3. Pour into mugs and add honey and lemon as desired.

4. Store the loose tea in a cool, dry place out of direct sunlight for up to 1 year.

Immunity Balls

This recipe is a take on Rosemary Gladstar's Zoom Balls, but in this version, herbs are used to stimulate and support the immune system. You can substitute almost any ingredient to your taste preferences or needs. For instance, you can use sunflower seed butter if nuts are a problem. Eat a couple of these a day during flu season for a tasty, nutritious, immunity-boosting snack.

MAKES 48 (1-INCH) BALLS

1 cup cashew, almond, or peanut butter

½ cup raw honey or blackstrap molasses

¼ cup astragalus root powder

¼ cup calendula powder

¼ cup echinacea root powder

¼ cup holy basil powder

½ cup cocoa powder, divided (optional)

1 tablespoon ground ginger

1 tablespoon ground cardamom

1 tablespoon ground cinnamon

½ cup shredded coconut (optional)

1. In a large bowl, using a large spoon, mix together the nut butter and honey.

2. Gradually add the astragalus, calendula, echinacea, and holy basil powders; ¼ cup of cocoa powder (if using); and the ginger, cardamom, and cinnamon to the mixture to form a stiff dough.

3. Roll into bite-size balls. If desired, roll them in the remaining ¼ cup of cocoa powder and/or shredded coconut.

4. Store in the refrigerator in a labeled, dated, air-tight container for up to 6 months, or 2 weeks at room temperature.

Spicy Chai

It is well worth gathering all the delicious spices for this sweet, warm, and rich beverage. Each ingredient is packed with health benefits and healing powers, and the combination packs a big flavor punch. This is the perfect hot drink for the cooler months.

MAKES 4 CUPS

3 slices fresh ginger

6 whole cloves

1 (3-inch) cinnamon stick, broken into small pieces

1 tablespoon dried holy basil

½ teaspoon coriander seeds

3 whole peppercorns

3 cardamom pods

½ teaspoon fennel seeds

3 black tea bags

3 cups cold water

6 to 8 tablespoons half-and-half

2 tablespoons raw honey

In a medium saucepan, gently warm the ginger, cloves, cinnamon, holy basil, coriander seeds, peppercorns, cardamom, fennel seeds, tea bags, water, half-and-half, and honey over low heat, covered, for 10 to 15 minutes. Do not let the mixture boil. Strain into a teapot. Compost the solids. Serve.

Tonic Soup

Warming and delicious, this soup gives you an immunity boost. It freezes well, so it's easy to keep on hand through the winter. There's nothing like soup to keep the chills away.

CONTINUED »

SERVES 8

8 cups beef, chicken, or
vegetable broth
1 tablespoon olive oil
1 onion, diced
4 to 8 garlic
cloves, minced
1 (1-inch) piece fresh
ginger, peeled and
finely chopped
1 cup sliced carrot
1 cup chopped fresh
burdock root (sold
in stores as gobo) or
sweet potatoes
2 pieces dried chopped
(cut and sifted)
astragalus root
1 cup sliced shiitake
mushrooms (fresh
or reconstituted)
3 cups chopped kale or
collard green leaves
(½-inch pieces)

1. In a large pot over high heat, bring the broth
   to a boil.

2. Meanwhile, in a large skillet, heat the olive oil
   over medium heat. Add the onion, garlic, and
   ginger. Reduce the heat to low and sauté until soft
   and fragrant.

3. Add the contents of the skillet to the broth in the
   pot, along with the carrot, burdock root, astragalus
   root, and mushrooms.

4. Simmer, covered, over low heat for 50 minutes.

5. Add the greens and simmer for 10 minutes more.

6. Remove the astragalus with a fork or tongs
   before serving.

7. Refrigerate leftovers for up to 1 week, or freeze in a
   labeled, dated, airtight container for 3 to 4 months.

IMMUNITY ISSUES

Turmeric Spice Nightcap

*This version of golden milk is a delicious treat to drink in the evening and
imparts all the glorious health benefits of turmeric and ginger. Turmeric in
particular is activated when mixed with black pepper and fats.*

CONTINUED »

2 cups water

4 ounces fresh turmeric root, grated (wear gloves for this)

1 (1-inch) piece fresh ginger, grated

1 tablespoon ground cinnamon

2 teaspoons freshly ground black pepper

½ teaspoon ground nutmeg

3 teaspoons coconut oil

1 cup milk of your choice (dairy, soy, or nut)

1 heaping teaspoon raw honey

1. In a large saucepan over high heat, bring the water to a boil.

2. Reduce the heat to low and bring the water to a simmer.

3. Add the turmeric, ginger, cinnamon, pepper, nutmeg, and coconut oil and stir while simmering for a few more minutes, or until the liquid forms a paste.

4. In another saucepan, warm the milk over low heat.

5. Pour the warmed milk into a mug. Add a heaping teaspoon of the paste and the honey. Stir to mix well before drinking.

6. The leftover paste will keep in a labeled, dated, airtight jar in the refrigerator for up to 2 weeks.

INFERTILITY

Adaptogen Nuggets

Maca is a root vegetable that has been used as an aphrodisiac to boost fertility and sex drive for centuries. Traditionally, this "Peruvian ginseng" was taken for increased energy and stamina. Maca has been known to restore hormonal balance. Adding ashwagandha can also increase sperm count.

CONTINUED »

MAKES ABOUT 100 NUGGETS (1½ TEASPOONS EACH)

1 cup almond butter, plus more as needed

¼ cup tahini

½ cup raw honey, plus more as needed

2 tablespoons raw cacao powder

1 tablespoon ground cinnamon

¼ cup coconut flakes

2 tablespoons dried holy basil

¼ cup astragalus root powder

2 tablespoons ashwagandha root powder

2 tablespoons maca powder

1 tablespoon gotu kola powder

1. In a medium bowl, combine the almond butter and tahini and mix well.

2. Add the honey, cacao, cinnamon, and coconut and mix thoroughly.

3. Mix in the holy basil, astragalus, ashwagandha, maca, and gotu kola. Add more honey or almond butter as needed to hold the mixture together well.

4. Break the dough into 1-inch sections and shape into small squares with your hands.

5. Place the dough squares in the refrigerator for at least an hour to firm up before enjoying.

6. Store in a tightly sealed, labeled, and dated container and eat within 2 weeks. These can also be stored in the refrigerator for up to 1 month.

INFERTILITY

Shatavari Fertility Elixir

Shatavari is one of the best herbs for reproductive health. It has no toxic side effects and may help improve overall fertility.

CONTINUED »

The adaptogens in this elixir are specifically aimed at supporting women's reproductive health. Lowering stress is also an important part of a holistic plan for fertility, and these adaptogens are perfect, since they can help your body and mind adjust to stressful situations.

MAKES 2 SERVINGS

2 cups almond milk or
    gluten-free oat milk
1 teaspoon maca powder
1 teaspoon shatavari
    root powder
1 tablespoon raw
    cacao powder
1 teaspoon
    ashwagandha
    root powder
2 teaspoons tahini
2 teaspoons raw honey
¼ teaspoon
    ground cinnamon

1. In a medium saucepan, warm the almond milk over low heat.

2. Whisk in the maca, shatavari, cacao, and ashwagandha until thoroughly mixed.

3. Whisk in the tahini and honey.

4. Transfer to a blender and blend for 20 seconds for a creamy and frothy drink. Top with cinnamon before serving.

5. Store leftovers in the refrigerator in a labeled, dated container for up to 2 days.

INSECT BITES AND STINGS

Honey-Lavender Compress

Lavender essential oil, honey, and baking soda help remove the venom from bee stings and itchy insect bites. If you are allergic to bees or notice increased pain and swelling at the site of a sting, seek medical attention right away.

MAKES 1 COMPRESS

2 teaspoons raw honey

1 teaspoon olive oil
7 drops lavender
    essential oil

½ teaspoon baking soda

CONTINUED »

1. In a small bowl, combine the honey, olive oil, lavender oil, and baking soda and mix well.

2. Apply the mixture to the affected area, cover the area with a 4-by-4-inch soft cloth, and apply an ice pack over the cloth. Leave the compress in place for 15 minutes, then rinse the area with cold water.

3. Repeat as needed to prevent pain and itching.

INSECT BITES AND STINGS

Relief Formula and Compress

When stung or bitten by an insect, I like to take a two-pronged approach: I'll apply the remedy directly to the afflicted area and take it internally as well. This allows the herbs to directly soothe the area while also supporting the body to reduce the histamine reaction.

MAKES 4 OUNCES

¼ **cup peach tincture**
2 **tablespoons**
  basil tincture
2 **tablespoons**
  echinacea tincture

1. In a 1-cup glass measuring cup, combine the peach tincture, basil tincture, and echinacea tincture and mix well.

2. Using a small metal funnel (if you have one) or a measuring cup with a spout, pour the tincture blend into a 4-ounce dropper bottle.

3. Tighten the dropper lid on the bottle and label with the name of the formula, the date, and the dosage information.

4. If you have been stung by a bee, be sure to carefully remove the stinger first by using a thin and rigid object such as a fingernail or credit card. Reverse the stinger out of the skin by pressing at

CONTINUED »

the edge of where the stinger is embedded. Soak a small piece of cloth in the tincture blend and apply it to the wound. Repeat every 20 to 30 minutes or when the cloth feels hot to the touch.

5. Separately, add 1 to 2 dropperfuls (25 to 50 drops) of the tincture blend into a small glass of water or juice and drink every 20 minutes for 1 to 2 hours, or until the swelling has reduced.

INSECT BITES AND STINGS

Tick and Spider Bite Poultice

Tick and spider bites can be scary because of the threat of Lyme disease from ticks and toxic bites from brown recluse spiders. It's always important to have a medical care practitioner check out the bites, but in the meantime, this poultice helps draw the toxins out of your body.

MAKES 1 POULTICE

1 or 2 fresh plantain leaves, or 1 teaspoon dried plantain leaf
30 drops echinacea tincture
10 drops peach tincture
1 teaspoon activated charcoal

1. For best results, chew the fresh plantain leaves until they are mashed into a poultice. This provides saliva, which helps with healing. If you do not want to chew the poultice, the leaves can be chopped finely and mixed with 1 tablespoon of boiling water, then drained after 15 minutes.

2. In a small bowl, mix the plantain with the echinacea tincture, peach tincture, and charcoal.

3. Apply directly over the bite and cover with an adhesive bandage. Repeat every 8 to 12 hours for up to 7 days or until the bite has healed.

Linden and Passionflower Elixir

I like to combine linden with passionflower to help with sleeplessness. Passionflower is specifically helpful for those times when thoughts go around and around in your head. The two herbs used together have a calming and sedative effect.

MAKES ABOUT 16 OUNCES

1½ cups brandy
½ cup raw honey
¾ cup dried linden
¾ cup dried
   passionflower
Juice and zest
   of 1 lemon

1. In a 24-ounce jar, combine the brandy and honey. Stir or cover and shake until the honey is dissolved.

2. Add the linden, passionflower, and lemon zest and juice, and mix very well. Cover, label, and date the jar.

3. Allow everything to steep for at least 1 month, shaking daily if possible.

4. Strain, then compost the solids. This can be stored in a cool, dry place out of direct sunlight for 5 years.

5. Use the elixir by the dropperful (25 drops). You can also add 1 teaspoon to 1 cup of tea or a small glass of plain brandy.

Sleepy Time Balm

Sleep balms are fun to make, and they only require a few ingredients. Essential oils such as lavender have been known to help people feel relaxed.

MAKES ABOUT 4¼ OUNCES

¼ cup coconut oil
1 tablespoon beeswax

1 teaspoon shea butter
   or cocoa butter
6 drops vetiver
   essential oil

6 drops lavender
   essential oil
6 drops lemon balm
   essential oil

CONTINUED »

1. In a double boiler, combine the coconut oil, bees-wax, and shea butter.

2. Heat the double boiler until the mixture is completely melted. Add the vetiver, lavender, and lemon balm essential oils and pour into small storage containers.

3. Allow the mixture to cool on the countertop.

4. When cool, cover, label, and date the containers. Store them in a cool, dry place and use within 6 to 9 months.

5. To use, put some balm on your fingers and then massage across the bottom of your feet and along your spine. It may seem greasy at first, but it will be absorbed quickly.

INSOMNIA

Sweet Dreams Herbal Tea Blend

Occasional insomnia happens to almost everyone. Soothe your mind and help your body relax with this wonderfully calming herbal tea blend. Make a large batch ahead of time so you always have some on hand when you need it.

MAKES 96 DOSES

1 cup dried
  chamomile flowers
1 cup dried
  passionflower

1 cup dried lemon balm
1 cup dried chopped
  (cut and sifted)
  valerian root

Raw honey or stevia, for
  sweetening (optional)

CONTINUED »

1. In a large bowl, combine the chamomile flowers, passionflower, lemon balm, and valerian root. Transfer to a labeled, dated glass container with a lid.

2. Use 2 teaspoons of the tea blend for every cup of boiling water, allowing the herbs to steep for 15 to 20 minutes before straining, composting the solids, and drinking the tea.

3. Sweeten with a little honey (if using).

4. Store the loose tea in a cool, dry place out of direct sunlight for up to 1 year.

5. Drink 1 cup 1 hour before bedtime.

IRRITABLE BOWEL SYNDROME (IBS)

Dandelion and Peppermint Tonic

We have things called bitter taste receptors located throughout our gastrointestinal tract, and when they're activated by bitter herbs and foods, they release the saliva, enzymes, and bile we need to break down food. Bitter foods, including dandelion and ginger, may assist in relieving IBS symptoms.

MAKES 1 SERVING

5 to 10 fresh
   peppermint leaves
1 (2-inch) piece fresh
   ginger, peeled and
   thinly sliced
5 to 10 fresh
   dandelion leaves
1 cup hot water

1. Slap the peppermint leaves between the palms of your hands to release their natural oils.

2. Gently pound the ginger slices on a cutting board with the back of your knife to release their natural juice.

3. Put the peppermint leaves, ginger, and dandelion leaves in the hot water.

CONTINUED »

4. Steep for about 10 minutes.

5. Strain and compost the solids before drinking the tea.

IRRITABLE BOWEL SYNDROME (IBS)

Gutsy Brew

If you're prone to IBS or any type of autoimmune issue that shows up in the gut, you may experience flare-ups during emotionally trying times. Of course, they can happen to anyone, so if discomfort becomes a problem, turn to this tea, which coats and soothes the gut and bowel. For this remedy, you use a cold infusion method, so it's best made up the night before you plan to drink it.

MAKES 1 QUART

1 tablespoon dried plantain leaf

1 tablespoon dried chopped (cut and sifted) marshmallow root

1 tablespoon dried rose petals

2 dried astragalus root slices

1 tablespoon dried peppermint

About 1 quart of cold water

1. In a 1-quart jar, combine the plantain, marshmallow root, rose, astragalus, and peppermint.

2. Fill the jar with cold water. Cover and label the jar.

3. Place the mixture in the refrigerator overnight.

4. In the morning, strain the liquid and compost the solids. Drink throughout the day. Leftover liquid can be stored in the refrigerator for up to 2 days.

Slippery Elm Tea

Slippery elm reduces inflammation and coats the intestinal lining. It also promotes regular bowel movements, both alleviating diarrhea and preventing constipation. This tea is a good remedy to try anytime you suffer from digestive upset.

MAKES 1 DOSE

2 cups boiling water

1 tablespoon slippery
  elm powder

1 tablespoon raw honey

1 teaspoon freshly
  squeezed lemon juice

1. In a large mug, combine the water, slippery elm powder, honey, and lemon juice. Allow the treatment to steep until it is cool enough to sip comfortably.

2. Drink a full mug of this tea 1 to 3 times a day for best results.

Aloe–Tea Tree Gel

Fresh aloe vera gel is a natural anesthetic and antifungal agent, making it perfect for treating jock itch. When you make this simple balm with aloe and tea tree oil, you'll enjoy instant relief and quick healing.

MAKES 5 DOSES

4 tablespoons fresh aloe
  vera gel

20 drops tea tree
  essential oil

1. In a small bowl, combine the aloe vera gel and tea tree oil.

2. Apply the balm to the affected area using your fingers or a cotton pad, allow it to air-dry, and put on a clean pair of cotton boxer shorts before

CONTINUED »

dressing. Use the balm as needed in the morning and evening until the condition clears.

3. Cover any leftover gel with plastic wrap, label the bowl and date it, and keep it in the refrigerator for up to 3 days.

Oregon Grape Gargle

This herbal gargle provides quick relief and is safe to use as often as needed to keep pain at bay. It may also be used for sore throats associated with colds and the flu.

MAKES 16 DOSES

1 ounce dried chopped (cut and sifted) Oregon grape root, or 2 ounces chopped fresh Oregon grape root
1 tablespoon slippery elm powder
2 cups water

1. In a medium saucepan, combine the Oregon grape root, slippery elm powder, and water and bring the mixture to a boil over medium-high heat.

2. Reduce the heat to medium-low and allow it to simmer for 10 to 15 minutes, or until the liquid has been reduced by about half.

3. Remove the saucepan from the heat and allow the mixture to cool until it is safe to handle, then strain into a jar with a tight-fitting lid, using the back of a spoon to extract the liquid from the herbs. Compost the solids. Label and date the jar.

4. Gargle with 1 to 2 tablespoons at a time. Repeat as often as necessary.

5. Keep the jar in the refrigerator for up to 1 week.

Raspberry Leaf Infusion

Raspberry leaf tea is a well-known remedy for menstrual cramps, and because it relaxes the muscles, it is also an excellent treatment for leg cramps. If you don't have access to whole raspberry leaves, you will find that commercially available raspberry leaf tea provides some relief.

MAKES 1 DOSE

5 fresh raspberry leaves
2 cups water
Raw honey or stevia,
  for sweetening

1. In a medium saucepan, combine the raspberry leaves and water and bring the mixture to a boil over medium-high heat.

2. Reduce the heat to medium-low and allow the infusion to simmer for 10 to 15 minutes, or until the liquid reduces by half.

3. Strain into a large mug and compost the solids.

4. Add the honey and allow the infusion to cool slightly before sipping.

5. Drink the infusion up to 3 times a day as needed.

Lice Lambaster Liquid

When lice enter a household, they make everyone miserable. This oil helps get rid of the lice by suffocating them, without the use of harsh chemicals that can be irritating to the scalp.

CONTINUED »

MAKES 4 OUNCES

2 tablespoons black
  walnut–infused oil
  (page 30)
2 tablespoons
  rosemary-infused oil
  (page 30)
2 tablespoons
  sage-infused oil
  (page 30)
2 tablespoons
  fennel-infused oil
  (page 30)

1. In a glass measuring cup, combine the black walnut–infused oil, rosemary-infused oil, sage-infused oil, and fennel-infused oil and mix well.

2. Pour into a 4-ounce bottle. Tighten the lid on the bottle and label with the name of the formula and the date made.

3. Apply a liberal amount of oil to the scalp and massage. Cover with a shower cap and leave on for 30 minutes, then use a lice comb to comb out the lice.

4. Rinse with warm water, then shampoo and rinse again. Repeat as needed. The remaining liquid can be stored in a cool, dry place out of direct sunlight and should be used within 1 year.

MENOPAUSE

Black Cohosh Decoction

Black cohosh has a bitter taste, but its benefits, which include reducing hot flashes, minimizing vaginal dryness, and stabilizing mood, make it an excellent choice for people suffering from typical menopause symptoms. The peppermint in this decoction helps mask black cohosh's flavor.

MAKES 1 DOSE

2 cups water
2 tablespoons dried
  chopped (cut
  and sifted) black
  cohosh root

2 tablespoons crumbled
  dried sage
2 tablespoons
  dried peppermint

Raw honey or stevia,
  for sweetening

CONTINUED »

1. In a medium saucepan, combine the water, black cohosh root, sage, and peppermint and bring the mixture to a boil over medium-high heat.

2. Reduce the heat to medium-low and allow the decoction to simmer for 15 to 20 minutes until reduced by half.

3. Remove the pan from the heat, cover it with a lid, and allow the mixture to rest for about 15 minutes.

4. Strain into a large mug, using the back of a spoon to press as much liquid from the herbs as possible. Compost the solids.

5. Add the honey before drinking.

6. Drink 1 cup a day for best results.

MENOPAUSE

Milky Oat Tincture

Milky oats make an unusually thick tincture. This is totally normal, and you'll get used to it—trust me. After the healing properties are pulled into the alcohol, the steeping tincture will look almost gruel-like. Use a dropper or two a day.

MAKES ABOUT 2 CUPS

1½ **cups fresh milky oats**
2½ **cups 150-proof rum, plus more as needed**

1. Place the oats and rum in a blender and puree until the mixture reaches a slushy consistency; add more alcohol if necessary to achieve this consistency.

2. Transfer the mixture to a large, labeled jar and let steep for 4 to 6 weeks.

CONTINUED »

3. After 4 to 6 weeks, strain the mixture well using a tincture press or by spooning it into a muslin bag and squeezing. Compost the solids.

4. Store the tincture in the large jar at room temperature. It will keep indefinitely.

MUSCLE PAIN

Sore Muscle Salve

Tight muscles knot, hurt, and can eventually start to spasm if you ignore the pain. One wrong move, and your neck, lower back, or calf muscle clenches and messes up your whole day. It's much better to be aware of your body's needs and respond during the early stages with this terrific, soothing salve.

MAKES 4 OUNCES

2½ tablespoons St. John's wort–infused olive oil

2½ tablespoons ginger-infused olive oil

2 tablespoons peppermint-infused olive oil

1 tablespoon beeswax pastilles

1. In a measuring cup, combine the St. John's wort–, ginger-, and peppermint-infused olive oils.

2. In a small saucepan or microwave-safe bowl, combine 2 tablespoons of the oil blend and the beeswax.

3. Heat the mixture slowly until the beeswax liquefies, either over medium-low heat on the stovetop or in 30-second increments in the microwave, stirring well in between. Add the remaining oil blend to the warmed beeswax mixture and stir well to combine.

4. Pour the mixture while it's still warm and liquid into a 4-ounce jar.

5. Label and date the salve.

6. Store the salve in a cool, dry place out of direct sunlight for up to 6 months.

Willow Bark Muscle Rub

Willow bark is an excellent internal remedy, and it is also an effective topical remedy for soothing sore muscles, particularly after a hard day of physical labor or a tough workout. This muscle rub should be made well in advance. When properly stored, it will keep indefinitely.

MAKES 40 DOSES

3 ounces chopped dried
  willow bark
1 dried habanero pepper
½ cup water
2 cups 95-percent
  rubbing alcohol

1. Put the willow bark and habanero pepper in a 1-quart mason jar with a tight-fitting lid. Add the water and grain alcohol, cap the jar, and put it in a cool, dark place. Leave it there for 6 to 8 weeks, swirling the herbs and alcohol once a day.

2. At the end of the curing period, strain into a large pitcher or bowl. With the back of a spoon, mash all the alcohol out of the herbs. Compost the solids.

3. Using a funnel, carefully transfer the liquid to a labeled, dark-colored glass bottle with a narrow neck, and store it in a cool, dark place.

4. Apply about 1 tablespoon to sore muscles with a soft cloth or a cotton pad, avoiding contact with the eyes and mucous membranes.

Lavender-Peppermint Bath Oil

Both lavender and peppermint essential oils are excellent herbal remedies for nausea. This simple bath oil has a wonderful aroma and may be used for a relaxing massage even when you're feeling just fine. People who are or might be pregnant should not use this remedy.

CONTINUED »

MAKES 16 DOSES

1 cup sweet almond oil

20 drops lavender
essential oil

6 drops peppermint
essential oil

1. Using a funnel, pour the almond oil into a dark-colored glass bottle, then add the lavender and peppermint essential oils. Label and date the bottle.

2. Cover and shake the bottle well before each use. For best results, add 1 tablespoon of the bath oil into a tub of warm water, and remain in the bathtub for at least 15 minutes. To enhance the antinausea effect, sip a cup of hot peppermint tea while soaking.

3. This oil will keep in a cool, dry place for up to 1 year.

NAUSEA

Personal Nasal Inhaler with Ginger and Peppermint

This personal nasal inhaler is convenient, as you can carry it in your purse or backpack. Whenever you feel nauseated from motion sickness, car sickness, or any other trigger, simply sniff it. You can buy the personal inhaler online.

MAKES 1 INHALER

2 drops peppermint
essential oil

2 drops ginger
essential oil

2 drops lemon
essential oil

Drop the essential oils into the cotton part of a personal nasal inhaler. Inhale deeply through your nose as needed.

Sap Infusion in Oil or Tincture

Make one or both of these ahead so they are ready whenever you need them! You can use the oil internally as is or make it into a healing and warming salve. The aromatic properties of pine are an added bonus with every use.

MAKES ABOUT ¾ CUP

For the oil

¼ **cup pine sap**
½ **cup olive oil or other oil of your choice**

For the tincture

¼ **cup pine sap**
½ **cup 150-proof rum**

To make the oil

1. In an 8- or 12-ounce jar, combine the pine sap and olive oil.

2. Place the jar in a warm place, such as a windowsill, and let steep for up to a month, shaking the jar daily if possible. Alternatively, if you're in a hurry, you can warm it in a double boiler for 2 to 4 hours, until the sap is completely dissolved into the oil.

3. Strain into a bottle, label and date it, and compost the solids. Use as needed. The oil usually lasts at room temperature for 1 year or more.

To make the tincture

4. In an 8- or 12-ounce jar, combine the pine sap and rum.

5. Place the jar in a warm place, such as a windowsill, and let steep for up to a month, shaking the jar daily if possible.

6. Strain into a bottle, label and date it, and compost the solids. Use as needed.

7. The tincture will keep at room temperature indefinitely.

Chamomile Compress

Because of chamomile's anti-inflammatory and antimicrobial properties, the herb is ideal for soothing the pain and irritation of pinkeye.

MAKES 2 COMPRESSES

1 cup boiling water
2 chamomile tea bags

1. In a medium bowl, pour the boiling water over the tea bags and allow them to steep for 5 minutes. Remove the tea bags from the water and let them cool until they can be handled.

2. Lie down and close your eyes. Place the tea bags over your eyes and leave them in place for 15 minutes.

3. Make this simple compress 2 or 3 times daily and apply it for up to 3 days.

4. If you don't see an improvement, or if your condition seems to be worsening, stop using the compress and call your doctor.

POISON IVY AND POISON OAK

Poison Ivy and Poison Oak Relief

Nothing is worse than a poison ivy rash when you're out in the hot sun trying to pull weeds. This spray helps soothe that itch while helping dry out the oils that are under the skin to heal the rash faster. For a quick fix on the itch, run the rash under extremely hot water, as hot as you can stand (but not hot enough to burn your skin), for about 30 seconds. You'll notice an intense surge of the itch, but then it will go away. This is extremely helpful at night for when you're trying to fall asleep. Follow up with a generous dose of this spray.

CONTINUED »

MAKES 4 OUNCES

½ ounce
  peppermint tincture
½ ounce
  jewelweed tincture
½ ounce
  echinacea tincture
½ ounce
  rosemary-infused
  vinegar
¼ cup water

1. In a 1-cup glass measuring cup, combine the peppermint tincture, jewelweed tincture, echinacea tincture, infused vinegar, and water and mix well.

2. Pour the tincture into a 4-ounce glass bottle with a spray-top lid.

3. Tighten the lid on the bottle and label with the name of the formula and the usage information. In a cool, dark place, this spray can keep indefinitely.

POISON IVY AND POISON OAK

Witch Hazel Compress

Liquid witch hazel reduces the itching, burning, and swelling associated with exposure to poison ivy, poison sumac, and poison oak, while aloe vera gel soothes and heals inflamed skin.

MAKES 4 COMPRESSES

4 tablespoons
  alcohol-free aloe
  vera gel
4 tablespoons
  alcohol-free witch
  hazel hydrosol

1. In a small bowl, mix together the aloe and witch hazel.

2. Apply the mixture liberally to the affected area. Cover it with a 4-by-4-inch soft cloth and apply an ice pack on top of the cloth. Leave the treatment in place for at least 15 minutes.

3. Repeat as needed to keep the itching and pain at bay.

Balance Tea Blend

I've blended this lovely tea to address some of the most annoying aspects of premenstrual syndrome, but please don't keep it hidden and only pull it out a few days each month. Instead, serve it anytime your spirit is flagging and causing physical symptoms.

MAKES 50 (1-CUP) SERVINGS

½ cup dried nettles

½ cup dried lemon balm

¼ cup dried catnip

¼ cup dried chopped
(cut and sifted)
mimosa bark

1 tablespoon
ground ginger

Raw honey, for
sweetening (optional)

Lemon, for
serving (optional)

1. In a large bowl, combine the nettles, lemon balm, catnip, mimosa bark, and ginger.

2. Transfer the loose tea blend to an airtight container. Label and date the blend.

3. To use, put 1 rounded teaspoon in an infuser and place it in a 10-ounce mug.

4. Cover with boiling water and let steep for 5 to 7 minutes. Remove the infuser.

5. Sweeten with honey and lemon (if using).

6. Store the loose tea in a cool, dry place out of direct sunlight for up to 1 year.

Ginger–Black Cohosh Tonic

This tonic provides a reprieve from the headaches and disrupted emotions that may tend to come before a period. Make a large batch in advance and keep it in the refrigerator for up to one week if you like; either reheat it or enjoy it over ice.

CONTINUED »

Ginger–Black Cohosh Tonic *continued*

MAKES 1 DOSE

2 cups water
2 tablespoons dried
  chopped (cut
  and sifted) black
  cohosh root
5 raspberry leaves, fresh
  or dried
1 tablespoon grated
  fresh ginger
Raw honey or stevia,
  for sweetening

1. In a medium saucepan, combine the water, black cohosh root, raspberry leaves, and ginger and bring the mixture to a boil over medium-high heat.

2. Reduce the heat to medium-low and allow the tonic to simmer for 15 to 20 minutes, until the liquid reduces by half.

3. Remove the pan from the heat, cover it with a lid, and allow it to rest for about 15 minutes.

4. Strain into a mug, using the back of a spoon to press as much liquid from the herbs as possible. Compost the solids.

5. Add the honey.

RESPIRATORY ILLNESS

Echinacea Elderberry Gummies

Kids love these. It can be tough to get everyone on board the immunity train, especially if they think something is medicine—but a spoonful of sugar can make all the difference. These herbs will go a long way toward keeping viruses at bay.

MAKES 64 (1-INCH) PIECES

Nonstick cooking spray
2 cups Elderberry Syrup
  (page 181)
¼ cup freshly squeezed
  lemon juice

1 cup chopped dried
  echinacea roots,
  leaves, and flowers

4 tablespoons
  unflavored
  powdered gelatin
5 tablespoons sugar

1. Lightly grease a square glass baking dish or 64 (1-inch) square silicone candy molds with cooking spray. Set aside.

CONTINUED »

2. In a medium saucepan, combine the elder syrup, lemon juice, and echinacea and simmer over low heat until the liquid is reduced by about half. Set aside to cool. Strain into a medium bowl and allow the liquid to cool to room temperature. Compost the solids.

3. In another saucepan, combine the cooled liquid with the gelatin and sugar. Cook over low heat, stirring often, until the gelatin and sugar dissolve completely, about 3 minutes. Skim any foam from the surface.

4. Pour the mixture into the prepared baking dish and refrigerate until the mixture sets, about 10 minutes.

5. Cut into 1-inch squares or remove the gummies from the molds. Store in a labeled, dated, airtight container at room temperature for 5 days or in the refrigerator for up to 2 weeks.

RESPIRATORY ILLNESS

Marseilles Vinegar

There are many variations to this vinegar, so feel free to improvise. All of these ingredients have spectacular healing properties. You can use the vinegar by the spoonful in a glass of water, or include it as an ingredient or seasoning in a meal.

CONTINUED »

MAKES ABOUT 1 QUART

2 tablespoons
dried thyme

2 tablespoons
dried rosemary

2 tablespoons
dried sage

2 tablespoons dried
lavender flowers

2 tablespoons
dried peppermint

2 tablespoons
chopped garlic

1 quart apple
cider vinegar

1. In a 1-quart glass jar, combine the thyme, rosemary, sage, lavender, peppermint, garlic, and vinegar. Label and date the jar. Cover and let steep in a cool, dark place for about 2 weeks, shaking daily.

2. When the steeping is finished, strain and return the vinegar to the jar. Compost the solids.

3. Store at room temperature for up to 6 months.

RESPIRATORY ILLNESS

Sage and Garlic Soup

This is a nourishing soup to help you fight a wet, drippy head cold or heavily productive respiratory infection. The garlic comes out to do the heavy lifting, and the sage backs it up all the way.

MAKES ABOUT 8 CUPS

Cloves from
1 head garlic, minced
or crushed

½ cup fresh sage leaves,
coarsely chopped

¼ cup fresh
thyme leaves

¼ cup fresh
parsley leaves,
coarsely chopped

2 teaspoons minced
fresh ginger

1 pinch cayenne pepper

6 cups chicken or
vegetable broth

6 large egg
yolks, beaten

Salt

Freshly ground
black pepper

CONTINUED »

1. In a large pot, combine the garlic, sage, thyme, parsley, ginger, cayenne, and broth and bring the mixture to a boil over high heat.

2. Reduce the heat to low and simmer, uncovered, for 25 minutes.

3. Add a splash of hot soup to the egg yolks, whisking constantly. Then, slowly pour the yolk mixture into the soup.

4. Season with salt and pepper before serving.

RINGWORM

Lavender–Tea Tree Toner

Tea tree essential oil is a powerful antifungal agent that clears ringworm rapidly. This toner can also be used for soothing minor wounds, including burns.

MAKES 10 DOSES

40 drops tea tree essential oil
10 drops lavender essential oil
⅝ cup apple cider vinegar

1. In a small, dark-colored glass bottle, combine the tea tree oil, lavender oil, and vinegar. Label and date the bottle.

2. Put 5 drops of the toner on a cotton ball and swab the patches of ringworm. Discard the cotton ball after use. Repeat twice daily until the ringworm clears.

3. The toner will keep in a cool, dark place for up to 1 year.

Ringworm Relief

Black walnut and calendula are top-notch for eliminating ringworm. They work within days of the first application, and this tincture is great to have on hand to reduce the skin fungus.

MAKES 1 OUNCE

¾ **ounce black walnut hull tincture**

¼ **ounce calendula tincture**

1. In a 1-cup glass measuring cup, combine the black walnut hull tincture and calendula tincture and mix well.

2. Pour the tincture into a 1-ounce glass dropper bottle.

3. Tighten the dropper lid on the bottle and label with the name of the formula and the dosage information.

4. Apply several drops directly to the ringworm and lightly massage. Repeat 1 to 2 times daily until all traces of the ringworm are gone.

Rosemary–Tea Tree Sinus Treatment

Sinus infections bring pain and pressure with them. Irrigating your nasal passageways is an excellent way to clear them, and adding healing essential oils helps eliminate the infection. You can also use this remedy anytime you're feeling congested due to a cold, the flu, or seasonal allergies.

CONTINUED »

MAKES 48 DOSES

20 drops rosemary
  essential oil
12 drops tea tree
  essential oil
1 cup fine sea salt
1½ cups water
  (per dose)

1. In a medium glass jar, combine the rosemary and tea tree essential oils with the salt. Seal the jar with a lid, then label and date it.

2. To treat the sinuses, combine 1 teaspoon of the mixture with the water, and stir well to dissolve the salt.

3. Use a neti pot to cleanse your sinuses twice a day until symptoms clear. Be sure to keep tissues within reach so you can blow your nose after each treatment.

4. Store the treatment in a cool, dark place for up to 2 years.

SINUS INFECTION

Sinus Saver Formula

When you need relief from sinus congestion and pain, this formula can help. The herbs help soothe inflamed membranes, dry up mucus, and reduce infection.

MAKES 4 OUNCES

2 tablespoons
  echinacea tincture
2 tablespoons
  basil tincture
2 tablespoons
  peach tincture
1 tablespoon
  raspberry tincture
1 tablespoon dried
  nettles tincture

1. In a 1-cup glass measuring cup, combine the echinacea tincture, basil tincture, peach tincture, raspberry tincture, and nettles tincture and mix well.

2. Pour the tincture into a 4-ounce glass dropper bottle.

3. Tighten the dropper lid on the bottle and label with the name of the formula and the dosage information.

4. Add 1 to 2 dropperfuls (25 to 50 drops) of the tincture blend to a small glass of water or juice. Drink up to 4 times daily until you are symptom-free for 24 hours.

SORE THROAT

Chamomile-Eucalyptus Gargle

Chamomile and eucalyptus help soothe sore, swollen throat tissue while preventing infection from worsening. Use this gargle at the first sign of a sore throat, and you'll find your symptoms are less painful; also, the duration of your illness may be shortened.

MAKES 12 TO 24 DOSES

2 tablespoons dried chamomile flowers, or 4 tablespoons fresh chamomile flowers

2 cups water

3 drops eucalyptus essential oil

1. In a medium saucepan, combine the chamomile and water and bring the mixture to a boil over medium-high heat. Reduce the heat to medium-low and allow the infusion to simmer for about 15 minutes.

2. Strain into a jar, using the back of a spoon to press as much liquid from the flowers as possible. Compost the solids.

3. Once the infusion has cooled to room temperature, add the eucalyptus essential oil to the jar, cap it tightly, and shake it well. Label and date the jar.

4. Gargle with 1 to 2 tablespoons 3 times or more a day until symptoms subside. Avoid swallowing the gargle, as it might cause stomach upset.

5. Store the gargle in the refrigerator for up to 1 week.

SORE THROAT

Sage and Lemon Honey

In this delicious concoction, the lemon and honey gradually meld into a light syrup, punctuated by the sage. It's tasty and good medicine. If you're an adventurous cook, substitute this for regular honey in baking and savory recipes.

CONTINUED »

MAKES 8 TO 10 OUNCES

2 lemons, thinly sliced
   and seeded
½ cup fresh sage leaves,
   finely chopped
¾ to 1 cup raw honey

1. In a pint jar, combine the lemon slices and sage leaves.

2. Pour the honey over the lemon and sage, completely covering them.

3. Poke around the mixture with a skewer to get all the air bubbles out.

4. Strain, cover, and refrigerate. Label and date the jar. Use by the spoonful in healing teas.

5. Store in the refrigerator for up to 1 year.

SORE THROAT

Sore Throat Soother

Whether it's caused by allergies, a virus, or bacteria, a sore throat is painful. This tea helps reduce inflammation, ease pain, and heal the throat.

MAKES 24 (1-CUP) SERVINGS

¼ cup dried
   raspberry leaves
¼ cup dried
   ginger pieces
¼ cup dried thyme
2 tablespoons
   dried basil
2 tablespoons
   dried sage
1 cup boiling water
Raw honey, for
   sweetening (optional)

1. In a small bowl, combine the raspberry leaves, ginger, thyme, basil, and sage. Transfer to an airtight container and label with the ingredients and instructions for use.

2. Steep 2 teaspoons of the tea blend in the boiling water for 15 to 20 minutes.

3. Add honey (if using) to sweeten.

4. Drink 1 cup as needed.

5. Store the loose tea in a cool, dry place out of direct sunlight for up to 1 year.

Throat Spray

This blend of soothing roots and bark is very effective for sore throats or for when your voice is scratchy or has vanished because of illness or overuse. One or two spritzes can provide immediate relief that lasts a good while, and the spray is safe to reuse often throughout the day.

MAKES 3 CUPS

1 quart water

1 tablespoon dried chopped (cut and sifted) licorice root

1 tablespoon dried chopped (cut and sifted) slippery elm bark

1 tablespoon dried chopped (cut and sifted) marshmallow root

1 tablespoon grated fresh ginger

1 cup 150-proof rum

1. In a large, heavy saucepan, combine the water and licorice root, slippery elm, marshmallow root, and ginger. Cover and soak overnight.

2. The following day, bring the mixture to a boil over medium-high heat and cook until the liquid is reduced by half (to about 2 cups).

3. Strain and compost the solids. Let the liquid cool completely.

4. Stir in the rum.

5. Pour the liquid into spray bottles, secure the spray tops, and use as needed. (I like to make and label several small bottles.)

6. Store in a cool, dark place indefinitely.

Splinter and Prickle Poultice

Splinters, glass slivers, and prickles can become embedded under the skin and hard to remove. This poultice helps draw them to the surface of the skin for easy removal. For deeply embedded splinters, expect to apply this poultice for up to a week to see results.

MAKES 1 POULTICE

1 or 2 fresh plantain
 leaves, or 1 teaspoon
 dried plantain leaf
30 drops peach tincture
1 teaspoon
 activated charcoal

1. For best results, chew the plantain leaves until they are mashed into a poultice. This provides saliva, which helps heal. If you do not want to chew the poultice, the leaves can be chopped finely and mixed with 1 tablespoon of boiling water, then drained after 15 minutes.

2. In a small bowl, mix the plantain with the tincture and charcoal.

3. Apply the poultice directly over the splinter and cover with an adhesive bandage. Repeat every 8 to 12 hours, until the splinter has come to the surface and can be removed with tweezers.

SOS Soak

SOS, in this case, stands for "sprains or strains," which can be excruciatingly uncomfortable. This soak helps reduce inflammation and repair damaged tissue while easing pain.

**MAKES 3 CUPS LOOSE TEA
(ENOUGH FOR 6 DOSES)**

1 cup dried
 raspberry leaves

1 cup chopped dried
 willow bark

CONTINUED »

½ **cup dried comfrey leaves**
½ **cup dried lavender flowers**
1 quart boiling water
2 tablespoons Epsom salts per dose

1. In a small bowl, combine the raspberry leaves, willow, comfrey, and lavender and mix well. Transfer to an airtight container and label with the date, ingredients, and instructions for use.

2. While boiling the water, put 2 tablespoons of Epsom salts and ½ cup of the herb blend in a heatproof plastic shoebox or tub. Add the boiling water to the shoebox and steep until the liquid has cooled enough to comfortably submerge any sore or strained extremity in it. Soak for 20 minutes.

3. Repeat the soak 2 to 3 times daily until the sprain or strain is healed.

4. Store the loose tea in a cool, dry place out of direct sunlight for up to 1 year.

SWIMMER'S EAR

Tea Tree Oil Ear Treatment

Though wonderfully simple, this tea tree oil ear treatment is a powerful remedy for swimmer's ear, as it dries out the infected area and kills bacteria that would otherwise multiply.

MAKES 1 DOSE

2 drops tea tree essential oil diluted in 1 teaspoon olive oil

1. Lie on your side with the affected ear up. Drip the diluted tea tree oil into the ear with an eyedropper. If you need to treat both ears, place a cotton ball in the already treated ear to keep the essential oil inside while you treat the second ear.

2. Repeat this treatment twice a day until symptoms clear.

Chamomile Ice Pops

Teething can be a painful ordeal for babies, and listening to your little one cry in pain can be heartbreaking. Chamomile ice pops help soothe the pain, bring down swelling, and calm the baby. The act of sucking on an ice pop can take baby's mind off the discomfort.

MAKES 8 ICE POPS

4 chamomile tea bags, 4 tablespoons dried chamomile flowers, or 8 tablespoons fresh chamomile flowers

4 cups water

1. Place the chamomile tea bags in a medium saucepan with the water and bring the mixture to a boil. Reduce the heat and allow the mixture to simmer for 10 to 15 minutes, until the liquid reduces by half.

2. Remove the saucepan from the heat and allow the mixture to cool completely, then strain and pour it into ice pop molds. Freeze the molds overnight or until solid.

Licorice Tooth Polish Powder

The ingredients in this tooth polish help clean stains and promote gum health. If you like the taste of licorice, then you're in for a tasty treat while cleaning! It is difficult to grind spices or roots into a nice powder, so it's best to purchase these ingredients already powdered.

MAKES ABOUT ½ CUP

¼ cup kaolin or bentonite clay

1 tablespoon baking soda

2 teaspoons fine sea salt

2 teaspoons licorice root powder

1 teaspoon activated charcoal powder

1 teaspoon ground peppermint

½ teaspoon ground cloves

½ teaspoon ground thyme

CONTINUED »

1. In a large jar, combine the kaolin or bentonite clay, baking soda, salt, licorice root, charcoal, peppermint, cloves, and thyme. Cover and shake to mix well. Label and date the jar.

2. Keep about 1 tablespoon of the polish mix in a small jar or container. Put a pinch of the mixture in the palm of your hand and pick it up with a wet toothbrush. Brush as you normally would and rinse well.

3. Keep the bulk of the mixture stored in the large jar (this way, if the small container gets wet, the whole batch won't be ruined).

4. Store the powder at room temperature for up to 2 years.

TEETH ISSUES

Sage-Salt-Soda Tooth Powder

This natural tooth powder will leave your teeth feeling clean, make your breath fresh, and whiten your teeth.

MAKES 1 CUP

½ **cup fresh sage leaves**
¼ **cup sea salt**
2 **tablespoons baking soda**

1. Using a mortar and pestle, grind the sage leaves into the sea salt.

2. Spread out the ground salt and sage in a glass baking dish, and put it in the oven. Turn your oven to the lowest possible setting and let the mixture heat for 1 to 2 hours, until it hardens.

CONTINUED »

3. Remove the dish from the oven, let the mixture cool until you can handle it, then spoon it back into the mortar and pestle and regrind. Add the baking soda and mix well.

4. Pour into an airtight container and label. Store the mixture in a cool, dry place out of direct sunlight for up to 1 year.

5. Wet your toothbrush, then sprinkle the mixture onto it. Brush your teeth as normal.

TEETH ISSUES

Tea Tree Toothache Rinse

Alcohol helps numb tooth pain, and tea tree essential oil kills the bacteria that can contribute to the pain. A periodontal infection can become serious quickly and cause irreversible bone damage if not treated appropriately. Be sure to see your dentist if the pain does not subside within two to three days or if severe swelling or a fever accompanies your toothache. Note: Do not use rubbing alcohol for this treatment, since that type of alcohol is toxic!

MAKES 4 TO 8 DOSES

½ **cup vodka**

16 **drops tea tree essential oil**

1. Mix the vodka and tea tree essential oil together in a jar, and label it.

2. Swish with 1 to 2 tablespoons 3 times daily, using your cheeks to hold the rinse near the affected tooth for up to 1 minute before spitting. Avoid swallowing the rinse, as it might cause stomach upset.

Calendula Infusion

Thrush is a painful condition that can disrupt a baby's feeding schedule. Calendula soothes the pain while killing the fungus that causes thrush. This infusion may also be spritzed onto diaper rash after the baby's bath and before applying a barrier cream. For adults, this infusion can help heal mild cases of athlete's foot, ringworm, and jock itch. If this treatment doesn't bring an improvement for your baby within three days, call the pediatrician to ensure that the thrush doesn't get worse.

MAKES ABOUT 2 CUPS

3 teaspoons dried
  calendula flowers,
  or 6 teaspoons fresh
  calendula flowers
2 cups water

1. In a medium saucepan, combine the calendula and water and bring the mixture to a boil over medium-high heat.

2. Reduce the heat to medium-low and allow the mixture to simmer for 10 to 15 minutes, or until the liquid reduces by half.

3. Strain into a jar, using the back of a spoon to press as much liquid from the flowers as possible. Compost the solids.

4. Cap the jar tightly and allow the infusion to cool at room temperature before using it. Prepare a fresh infusion daily.

THYROID IMBALANCE

Matcha Zen Latte

Stress can have a negative effect on your thyroid function. A common example of chronic stress is adrenal fatigue, which occurs when your adrenal glands are unable to keep up with physiological needs. One way to combat this is to

CONTINUED »

reduce coffee consumption. Replace it with a matcha green tea latte, which contains L-theanine, an amino acid that reduces cortisol and helps you feel calmer. Try adding adaptogenic herbs to your drinks. Adaptogens have been shown to decrease levels of cortisol, a stress hormone secreted when our body experiences stress.

MAKES 1 SERVING

½ to 1 teaspoon matcha green tea powder

½ cup hot water (just below boiling)

½ to 1 cup coconut milk, oat milk, or almond milk

1. For the best texture, whisk the matcha green tea powder with the hot water using a bamboo whisk in a small round bowl. This breaks up any clumps and will make the latte taste creamier. A stainless-steel whisk would also work.

2. Pour the matcha mixture into your favorite mug. Whisk until dissolved.

3. Heat the coconut milk on the stovetop or in a frothing pitcher.

4. Pour the milk into your mug and enjoy immediately.

TREMORS

Passionflower or Skullcap Electuary

Passionflower is a powerful herbal remedy that helps improve the levels of gamma-aminobutyric acid (GABA) in the brain, which works to lower over-active brain activity. Because of this effect, it can also help reduce essential tremors. An electuary is basically a powdered herb mixed with raw honey. This preparation has been used for centuries and helps make the herbs more palatable and long-lasting. The texture can be similar to a syrup or a thick paste.

CONTINUED »

**MAKES ABOUT 10 SERVINGS
(18 TEASPOONS)**

2 tablespoons powdered
    passionflower
    or skullcap
¼ cup raw honey
1 cup warm water
    (per dose)

1. Place the skullcap in a small bowl. Add enough honey to create a thick paste. Mix thoroughly.

2. Store the paste in an airtight glass container, such as a mason jar, for up to 1 year. Label and date the jar.

3. As needed, scoop out 1 to 2 teaspoons of the paste and add to the cup of warm water. Steep the tea for 10 minutes and drink.

ULCERS

Calendula Tea

Calendula eases the pain and burning associated with stomach ulcers by protecting the stomach's lining and reducing inflammation while acting as an antibacterial agent. If you have an ulcer that doesn't respond to treatment with herbal medicine within about a week, seek medical attention.

MAKES 1 DOSE

1 tablespoon dried
    calendula flowers, or
    2 tablespoons fresh
    calendula flowers
2 cups water
Raw honey or stevia, for
    sweetening (optional)

1. In a medium saucepan, combine the calendula and water and bring the mixture to a boil over medium-high heat. Reduce the heat to medium-low and allow the mixture to simmer for about 10 minutes.

2. Strain into a large mug and compost the solids. Allow the tea to cool slightly.

3. Add a little honey (if using) to sweeten.

4. Drink the entire dose 3 times a day, continuing for at least 2 weeks after symptoms have subsided.

Horseradish Vodka

You can use this as the alcohol in a Bloody Mary or mix it with just a swallow of juice to get its healing benefits. This recipe is a good way to preserve fresh horseradish instead of making a ton of cocktail sauce or jars of horseradish mixed in vinegar.

MAKES 1 QUART

1 (8-inch) piece fresh
  horseradish root,
  finely grated
3 cups 100-proof vodka

1. Let the grated horseradish rest for about 10 minutes to allow the oils to release and the "heat" to develop.

2. Put the horseradish in a 1-quart bottle and pour in the vodka. Close tightly and label.

3. Before using, give the bottle a good shake (no need to strain). Use the horseradish vodka in a mixed drink or as a dose of medicine.

4. Store in a cool, dark place. Unless it's in a brown glass bottle, light will slowly lessen the heat of the horseradish; otherwise, it would last for a decade at least. If it is stored away from light, it will be good forever.

Uva Ursi UTI Decoction

Uva ursi is an excellent remedy for urinary tract infections; it contains a high level of vitamin C and is a natural antibacterial and antimicrobial agent. If your UTI doesn't start responding to herbal treatments within two days, see your doctor. Left untreated, a UTI can travel into the bladder and kidneys, causing a systemic infection that can be deadly.

CONTINUED »

MAKES 1 DOSE

2 teaspoons dried
    uva ursi leaves, or
    4 teaspoons fresh uva
    ursi leaves
2 cups water
Stevia, for sweetening
    (optional)

1. In a medium saucepan, combine the uva ursi leaves and water and bring the mixture to a boil over medium-high heat. Reduce the heat to medium-low and simmer for 15 to 20 minutes, until the liquid reduces by half.

2. Remove the saucepan from the heat and allow the decoction to cool before drinking. Add the stevia (if using) to mask the taste, but don't use honey or sugar, since avoiding sugar for the duration of a UTI can help speed healing.

3. Drink the entire dose. Repeat this remedy 3 to 4 times daily for up to 5 days.

YEAST INFECTION

Goldenseal-Tea Tree Poultice

Goldenseal, tea tree oil, calendula, and thyme come together in this useful yeast-infection poultice to soothe itching and stinging while killing harmful bacteria. If your symptoms do not begin to subside within two to three days of beginning this treatment, consult a doctor. Other illnesses sometimes have symptoms similar to those of a yeast infection.

MAKES ABOUT 24 DOSES

2 teaspoons
    goldenseal tincture
4 teaspoons thyme
    tincture
4 teaspoons calendula
    tincture
7 drops tea tree
    essential oil
1 teaspoon water
    (per dose)

1. In a dark-colored bottle, combine the goldenseal, thyme, and calendula tinctures with the tea tree essential oil. Cap, label, and date the bottle.

2. To use, in a small bowl, combine ½ teaspoon of the treatment with the water. Soak 1 tampon in the mixture. Insert the tampon and leave it in place for 1 hour, then remove it. Repeat the treatment every 12 hours until the yeast infection disappears.

3. Store the treatment in a cool, dark place for up to 1 year.

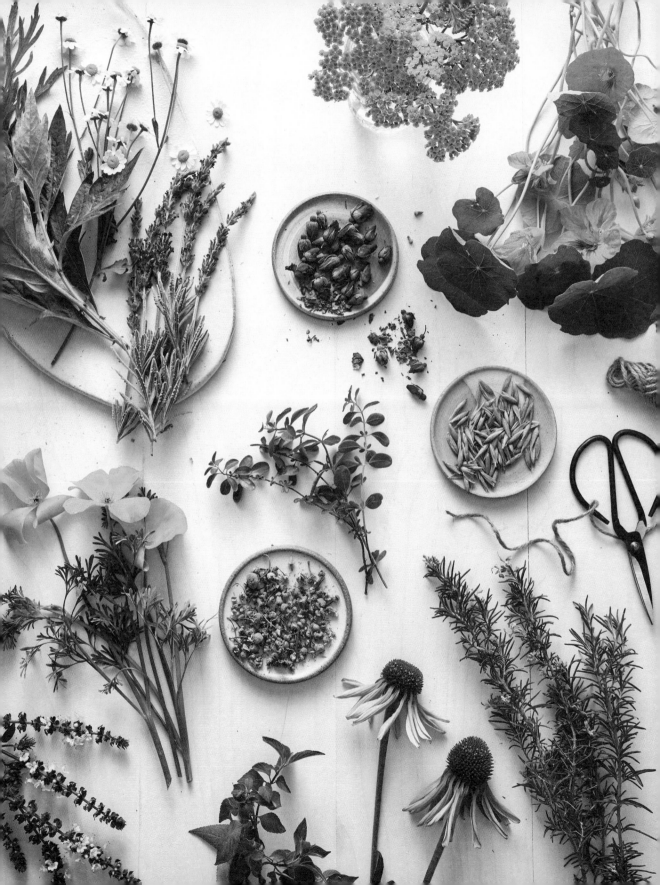

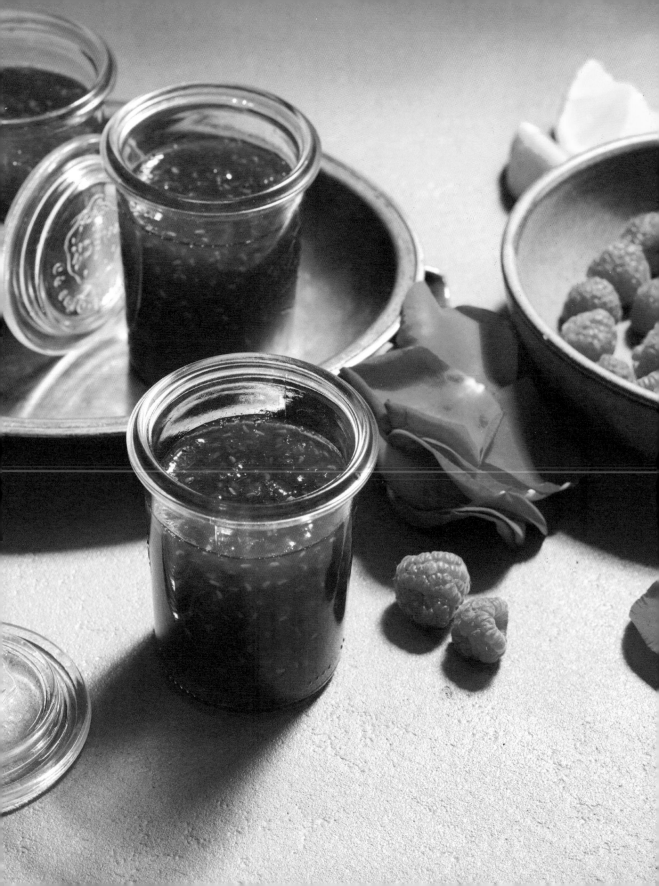

CHAPTER SIX

Remedies for Mental Health and Wellness

It can be surprising to find how important it is to "keep our spirits up." The mind-body connection is intricate, and it's impossible to be healthy in your body if your mind is ailing, and vice versa. We most often ignore our mental state because it's harder to see. Herbs can make a huge difference, and there are a wide range of remedies in this chapter that address most of the symptoms that can show up when we aren't at our best. Never hesitate to ask for help if you're hurting. Fixing the symptoms doesn't always fix the problem, whether mental, physical, emotional, or spiritual.

Calming Chamomile Lemonade

Chamomile tea is a well-known herbal remedy for children with ADD and ADHD. Serve this everyday treat over ice or make it into ice pops for a special sugar-free dessert.

MAKES 6 TO 12 DOSES

6 cups water
4 chamomile tea bags
Juice of 3 lemons
Stevia, for sweetening

1. In a large saucepan, boil the water over high heat. Add the tea bags and steep them in the boiling water for 15 minutes.

2. After removing the tea bags from the water, allow the tea to cool. Add the lemon juice and stevia, then transfer the lemonade to a pitcher, cover it, and chill it in the refrigerator. Label and date the pitcher.

3. Children under 5 years old should drink ½ cup per day; 5- to 12-year-old children should drink 1 cup a day. Teens and adults will benefit from 2 to 3 cups a day.

4. Store in the refrigerator for up to 1 week.

Ginseng-Spice Iced Tea

Ginseng can boost dopamine levels, help you focus, and improve your memory.

MAKES 1 GALLON

8 tablespoons dried chopped (cut and sifted) ginseng root

2 whole cinnamon sticks
5 whole cloves
1 tablespoon grated fresh ginger

8 cups water
Raw honey or stevia, for sweetening (optional)

CONTINUED »

1. In a large saucepan, combine the ginseng root, cinnamon, cloves, ginger, and water and bring the mixture to a boil over medium-high heat. Remove from the heat and allow the herbs to steep for 15 minutes.

2. Strain into a pitcher, using the back of a spoon to press the excess liquid from the herbs. Compost the solids. Label and date the pitcher.

3. Cool to room temperature.

4. Sweeten with honey (if using). Serve over ice.

5. Drink 2 to 4 glasses of tea daily, during the morning and early afternoon hours. Cut back if you have trouble sleeping.

6. Store in the refrigerator for up to 1 week.

ADDICTION AND SUBSTANCE ABUSE

Dandelion Tonic

Help your liver, kidneys, and spleen heal while clearing toxins with this simple tonic. Its taste is smooth, mellow, and mild, and drinking it will help you feel better.

MAKES 1 DOSE

2 teaspoons dried chopped (cut and sifted) dandelion root

1½ cups water

2 teaspoons raw honey

1. In a small saucepan, combine the dandelion root, water, and honey and bring the mixture to a boil over medium-high heat.

2. Reduce the heat to medium-low and simmer for 15 minutes.

CONTINUED »

3. Strain into a mug and compost the solids. Allow to cool slightly.

4. Drink this tonic daily while recovering from substance abuse.

ADDICTION AND SUBSTANCE ABUSE

Licorice–Milk Thistle Tonic

When recovering from an addiction, whether to junk food, cigarettes, alcohol, or drugs, it is important to support the body, mind, and spirit. Milk thistle contains silymarin, a combination of three antioxidants that helps reduce overall inflammation, so your body feels better while regaining balance. If you are taking Ativan, Orfidal, or another detoxification drug, be sure to talk to your doctor about potential interactions before using this remedy.

MAKES 1 DOSE

2 cups water
4 thin slices dried
   licorice root
1 to 2 dropperfuls
   (25–50 drops)
   standardized milk
   thistle extract
   (preferably liquid)
Raw honey or stevia, for
   sweetening (optional)

1. In a medium saucepan, combine the water and licorice root and bring the mixture to a boil over medium-high heat.

2. Reduce the heat to low and allow the mixture to simmer for 15 to 20 minutes, or until the liquid reduces by half.

3. Remove the pan from the heat, cover it with a lid, and allow the licorice root to rest for about 15 minutes.

4. Strain into a large mug, using the back of a spoon to press as much liquid from the herbs as possible. Compost the solids.

5. Stir in the milk thistle extract and a little honey (if using).

6. Drink the entire dose. Repeat the treatment up to 3 times daily.

Milk Thistle Liver Support

Enjoy this support as part of a complete detox. The silymarin in milk thistle protects and repairs liver cells while reducing inflammation.

MAKES 1 TREATMENT

20 drops milk
   thistle extract
1 tea bag (any flavor)
1 cup boiling water

1. In a mug, combine the milk thistle extract, tea bag, and boiling water.

2. Steep for 5 minutes.

3. Drink 4 cups per day before meals and snacks.

4. Use this remedy for 1 to 2 weeks while detoxifying your body.

Roasted Dandelion Kudzu "Coffee"

Kudzu, a Chinese medicinal herb, can help curb cravings, and dandelion root can aid in liver detoxification. This beverage is naturally rich and deliciously sweet, with a flavor similar to coffee. You can either gather dandelion roots from your garden or the wild, or buy the premade powder from a health-food store.

MAKES 1 DOSE

1½ teaspoons
   kudzu powder
2 tablespoons water,
   plus 2 cups

1 to 2 teaspoons roasted
   dandelion root powder
Pinch sea salt
Milk of choice, for
   serving (optional)

Raw honey or stevia, for
   sweetening (optional)

CONTINUED »

1. In a small bowl, dissolve the kudzu powder in 2 tablespoons of water and set aside.

2. In a medium saucepan, combine the dandelion root powder and the remaining 2 cups of water and simmer over medium heat for 10 minutes.

3. Add the sea salt and the kudzu mixture.

4. Continue simmering for another minute until the mixture thickens.

5. Drink as is or with a splash of milk (if using). Drizzle in a sweetener of your choice and blend to create a smooth, frothy latte. A blender or immersion blender would work for this.

ADDICTION AND SUBSTANCE ABUSE

St. John's Wort–Lemon Balm Tea Blend

Although we do not often compare herbs to pharmaceuticals, St. John's wort is sometimes referred to as "nature's Prozac." St. John's wort boosts your brain's serotonin levels, lifting your mood and bringing some relief from the effects of withdrawal. The lemon balm imparts an uplifting fragrance.

MAKES 120 (1-CUP) SERVINGS

1½ cups dried St. John's wort
1 cup dried lemon balm
1 cup boiling water

Raw honey or stevia, for sweetening (optional)

CONTINUED »

1. In a medium container, combine the St. John's wort and lemon balm. Seal, label, and date the container.

2. To use, put 1 teaspoon of the herb mixture in an infuser and place it in a 10-ounce mug. Pour the boiling water into the mug and let the tea steep for about 10 minutes. Remove the infuser.

3. Add the honey (if using) to sweeten.

4. Drink 2 cups of this tea each day.

5. Store the loose tea in a cool, dry place out of direct sunlight for up to 1 year.

AGITATION

Calm Candy

Although there is a lot of heat involved, the properties of these herbs still come through. Children love this candy, and it is convenient to take along almost anywhere. It's much easier to convince a non-herbal person to try a calming piece of candy than a dropperful of tincture.

MAKES 200 TO 300 PIECES OF CANDY (DEPENDING ON SIZE)

For the infusion

1½ cups water
¼ cup fresh passionflower, or 2 tablespoons dried passionflower

¼ cup fresh lemon balm, or 2 tablespoons dried lemon balm
¼ cup fresh chamomile flowers, or 2 tablespoons dried chamomile flowers
Juice and zest of 2 lemons

For the candy

2 tablespoons butter, divided
3 cups granulated sugar
¼ cup light corn syrup
Powdered sugar or cornstarch, for coating

CONTINUED »

To make the infusion

1. In a quart jar, combine the water, passionflower, lemon balm, chamomile, and lemon juice and zest. Seal it and allow it to sit overnight.

2. Strain into a clean pint jar and compost the solids.

To make the candy

3. Grease a large baking dish with 1 tablespoon of butter. Set aside.

4. Measure 1 cup of the infusion (but ¾ cup is enough—don't add water if there isn't a full cup).

5. In a medium saucepan, combine the measured infusion with the granulated sugar, corn syrup, and the remaining 1 tablespoon of butter. Heat over medium-high heat until the sugar dissolves.

6. Place a candy thermometer on the side of pan. Boil to exactly 300°F, with as little stirring as possible. (If the candy is not heated to 300°F, it will adhere to teeth and dental work.)

7. Remove the pan from the heat and pour the hot mixture into the prepared baking dish.

8. As soon as the candy cools enough to be handled, cut it into pieces and sprinkle with confectioner's sugar to keep pieces from sticking together.

9. Eat a piece of candy when you might otherwise have a cup of relaxing tea.

10. Store in a labeled jar in a cool, dry place for 6 months to 1 year. Despite being coated, the candy may still stick together after sitting in the jar. Vigorously shake or bump the jar against the counter (careful not to break the jar) to break up the pieces again.

Calming Cinnamon Tea

When life's pressures become overwhelming and you're feeling agitated, this calming cinnamon tea can help. With passionflower, hops, catnip, and cinnamon bark, it works wonders on frayed nerves and helps restore mental balance. This tea makes some people quite sleepy. Be sure to check your reaction to it before doing tasks that require your full attention.

MAKES 60 DOSES

1 cup chopped dried
   cinnamon bark (aka
   cinnamon chips)
¼ cup dried hops
¼ cup dried catnip
¼ cup dried
   passionflower
2 cups dried
   chamomile flowers

1. In a large container, combine the cinnamon bark, hops, catnip, passionflower, and chamomile flowers. Seal, label, and date the container.

2. To use, put 1 tablespoon in a tea infuser or strainer and steep in a mug of boiling water for 15 to 20 minutes. Remove the infuser and compost the solids.

3. Drink no more than twice a day.

4. Store the loose tea in a cool, dry place out of direct sunlight for up to 1 year.

Stop the World Elixir

This remedy is very good for that "last nerve" feeling we all get, and it has become a favorite of my friends for menopausal irritability.

MAKES ABOUT 1 QUART

½ cup dried
   borage flowers

½ cup dried holy basil
½ cup dried mimosa
   bark and flower
¼ cup dried motherwort

1 tablespoon dried
   lavender flowers
1 cup raw honey
4 cups vodka

CONTINUED »

1. In a half-gallon jar, combine the borage, holy basil, mimosa, motherwort, and lavender. Add the honey and mix well to coat the herbs.

2. Cover with vodka and mix well to be sure there are no air pockets.

3. Cover and infuse for 4 to 6 weeks.

4. Strain into a bottle and compost the solids. Label the bottle with the date, ingredients, and instructions for use.

5. Take 1 to 2 dropperfuls (25 to 50 drops) as needed. Alternatively, add up to ½ ounce to juice or a soft drink, or as part of the alcohol in a cocktail.

6. Store in a cool, dark place. This elixir can keep for at least 1 year.

ALZHEIMER'S DISEASE AND DEMENTIA

Peppermint-Ginkgo Infusion

Whole ginkgo is widely recognized for its ability to increase blood flow to the brain. This infusion may help enhance cognitive activity and reduce Alzheimer's and dementia symptoms. Be sure to talk with your health-care provider about using this infusion alongside conventional therapies to avoid possible adverse interactions. For best results, drink this infusion daily.

MAKES 1 DOSE

2 cups water

1 ounce crumbled dried ginkgo leaves

½ ounce crumbled dried peppermint

Raw honey or stevia, for sweetening

CONTINUED »

1. In a medium saucepan, combine the water, ginkgo, and peppermint and bring the mixture to a boil over medium-high heat.

2. Reduce the heat and allow the infusion to simmer for 10 to 15 minutes, or until the liquid reduces by half.

3. Remove the pan from the heat and allow the infusion to cool.

4. Once it is cool enough to drink, strain into a large mug, using the back of a spoon to extract as much liquid from the herbs as possible. Compost the solids.

5. Add a little honey and enjoy. This infusion can also be served chilled or over ice.

6. Drink 1 cup daily for best results.

ANGER

Anger Chaser Tincture

We all have felt angry, and it's often something we try to hide or feel ashamed of feeling. I suppose that in order for all of us to live together in a peaceable society, we've made anger into an emotion that shouldn't be expressed, making it all the more difficult to handle. This soothing herbal blend can help cool things down.

MAKES 2 OUNCES

3 tablespoons blue vervain tincture

3 tablespoons skullcap tincture

2 tablespoons mimosa tincture

2 tablespoons water or juice (per dose)

CONTINUED »

1. In a 1-cup glass measuring cup, combine the blue vervain, skullcap, and mimosa tinctures.

2. Transfer the mixture into a 4-ounce dropper bottle.

3. Label and date the tincture blend.

4. Take 1 dropperful (25 drops) in the water or juice. Repeat the dose 30 minutes later if needed.

5. Store the tincture blend in a cool, dark place for up to 3 years.

ANGER

Peaceful Passionflower Infusion

Anger is a normal emotion everyone experiences from time to time. Though it's important to acknowledge this emotion and understand its cause, it is equally important not to let the emotion take over, as anger can completely erode your sense of well-being. Drink this infusion to restore emotional balance when angry.

MAKES 1 DOSE

2 cups water
2 tablespoons dried passionflower
2 tablespoons dried chamomile flowers
2 tablespoons dried St. John's wort flowers
1 drop lavender essential oil diluted in 1 teaspoon olive oil
Raw honey or stevia, for sweetening (optional)

1. In a medium saucepan, combine the water, passionflower, chamomile, and St. John's wort and bring the mixture to a boil over medium-high heat.

2. Reduce the heat to medium-low and allow the infusion to simmer for 10 to 15 minutes, or until the liquid reduces by half.

3. Strain into a large mug, using the back of a spoon to press as much liquid from the herbs as possible. Compost the solids.

CONTINUED »

4. Apply a small amount of the diluted lavender essential oil to each of your temples and inhale the vapors from the infusion as it cools.

5. Add honey (if using).

6. Drink the infusion when it reaches a comfortable temperature.

7. Drink 1 cup as needed. In times of trouble, prepare a double or triple batch of the infusion and drink it 2 to 3 times daily.

ANXIETY

Bergamot Smelling Salt

Bergamot calms nervousness, focuses the thoughts, and helps eliminate feelings of stress. This smelling salt can help improve your state of mind quickly.

MAKES 1 OUNCE

1 ounce coarse sea salt
20 drops bergamot
  essential oil

1. In a small glass jar, combine the sea salt with the bergamot essential oil.

2. Cap tightly and shake well to blend.

3. Inhale deeply for 20 seconds. Store in a cool, dark place in between uses for up to 1 year.

4. Use this remedy as often as you like to ease anxiety and refocus your mind. Refresh the salt with additional essential oil when the fragrance begins to fade.

ANXIETY

Chamomile-Ginger Tea with Licorice

When focus and calm are what you need, look to chamomile, ginger, and licorice to keep nervousness and racing thoughts at bay. The sweet, spicy flavor of this tea makes it a delicious option as an everyday drink. Omit the licorice root in this recipe if you have high blood pressure.

MAKES 1 CUP

1 tablespoon dried
    chamomile flowers
1 teaspoon grated
    fresh ginger
1 teaspoon dried
    chopped (cut and
    sifted) licorice root
1¼ cups water

1. In a small saucepan, combine the chamomile, ginger, licorice, and water and bring the mixture to a boil over medium-high heat.

2. Reduce the heat to medium-low and simmer for 15 minutes.

3. Strain into a mug, using the back of a spoon to press the excess liquid from the herbs. Compost the solids.

4. Drink the tea anytime you are feeling anxious. Enjoy it as often as you like.

ANXIETY

Mask Refreshing Spray

Wearing face masks during contagious illnesses can make people who aren't accustomed to wearing them for work (like doctors and nurses) uncomfortable, including feeling claustrophobic. This spray does not completely sanitize, but it effectively removes the stale smell that develops from breathing through the mask. This should not replace regular laundering of reusable masks.

CONTINUED »

MAKES 4 OUNCES

½ cup 95-percent
  rubbing alcohol
20 drops peppermint
  essential oil
10 drops rosemary
  essential oil
10 drops eucalyptus
  essential oil

1. In a 1-cup glass measuring cup, combine the alcohol, peppermint oil, rosemary oil, and eucalyptus oil.

2. Divide evenly among 4 (1-ounce) small spray bottles. The spray can be put in larger bottles, if desired.

3. Label with the ingredients, date, and instructions for use (because of the high alcohol content). Store in a cool, dark place for up to 1 year.

4. Use whenever the mask feels or smells stale. Remove it and spray once on the inside and once on the outside. Let dry for several minutes or longer if possible.

5. If this is a reusable cloth mask, wash daily.

6. Note: This spray has a high enough alcohol content to use as a hand sanitizer, but will be very drying to the skin, though still good in a pinch.

ANXIETY

Misophonia Honey Electuary

The term misophonia *may be unfamiliar, but it's shocking how many people have it. It is when the sounds that people make eating, clearing their throats, clicking a pen, humming, or making other innocent motions prompt feelings of rage beyond reason. It sounds like no big deal unless you have it. It is painful, scary, and infuriating, and it is a symptom of chronic anxiety. This sweet herbal paste is easy to take along with you as you go about your day and can either be eaten or added to hot water for an instant tea.*

CONTINUED »

MAKES ABOUT 6 OUNCES

4 tablespoons dried
  holy basil
4 tablespoons dried
  lemon balm
2 tablespoons
  dried motherwort
¾ cup raw honey, plus
  more as needed

1. In a coffee grinder, working with one herb at a time, powder the holy basil, lemon balm, and motherwort. Sift the herbs through a mesh strainer into a medium bowl to remove bits of stem.

2. Add the honey to the powdered herb mixture, a bit at a time, until the mixture forms a thick paste. Use more honey if you prefer a thinner mixture.

3. Transfer to a 6-ounce jar or a number of smaller jars.

4. Label and date the electuary.

5. Add ½ to 1 teaspoon of the electuary to hot water to make tea, or eat it right off a spoon up to 3 times a day.

6. Store in the refrigerator for up to 1 month.

ANXIETY

Restless Circular Thinking Tincture

Circular thinking is a pretty common symptom of anxiety. It can manifest as someone working through a problem, talking it through, and then starting all over from the beginning. Over and over again.

MAKES 2 OUNCES

2 tablespoons
  passionflower tincture
1½ tablespoons
  valerian tincture

1½ teaspoons
  lavender tincture

2 tablespoons water or
  juice (per dose)

CONTINUED »

1. In a 1-cup glass measuring cup, combine the passionflower, valerian, and lavender tinctures.

2. Transfer the mixture into a 4-ounce dropper bottle.

3. Label and date the tincture blend.

4. Take 1 dropperful (25 drops) in the water or juice. Repeat the dose 30 minutes later if needed. This can be used up to 3 times a day.

5. Store the tincture blend in a cool, dark place for up to 3 years.

ANXIETY

Rosemary-Mint Nerve Tonic

Rosemary has a fresh, uplifting scent, and it contains compounds that relax the mind and ease anxiety. Chamomile and mint add fragrance, flavor, and even more relaxing compounds to the tonic, making it ideal anytime you need to lighten your mental load.

MAKES 1 DOSE

2 cups water

2 tablespoons crumbled dried rosemary, or 4 tablespoons chopped fresh rosemary

2 tablespoons dried chamomile flowers, or 4 tablespoons fresh chamomile flowers

2 tablespoons dried peppermint, or 4 tablespoons fresh peppermint leaves

Raw honey or stevia, for sweetening (optional)

1. In a medium saucepan, combine the water, rosemary, chamomile, and peppermint and bring the mixture to a boil over medium-high heat.

2. Reduce the heat to medium-low and simmer for 15 to 20 minutes, or until the liquid reduces by half.

CONTINUED »

3. Strain into a large mug, using the back of a spoon to press as much liquid from the herbs as possible. Compost the solids.

4. Sweeten with the honey (if using).

5. Drink 1 cup up to 3 times a day.

ANXIETY

St. John's Wort Infusion with Borage Oil

Anxiety can rob you of sleep, cause you to lose focus, and prevent you from enjoying life to its fullest. Borage, St. John's wort, and hawthorn berries help eliminate stress and reduce anxiety while uplifting your mood.

MAKES 1 DOSE

2 cups water
1 teaspoon dried St. John's wort flowers
1 tablespoon dried hawthorn berries
Raw honey or stevia, for sweetening
1 (1,000 mg) borage oil capsule

1. In a medium saucepan, combine the water, St. John's wort, and hawthorn berries and bring the mixture to a boil over medium-high heat.

2. Reduce the heat to medium-low and allow the infusion to simmer for 15 to 20 minutes, or until the liquid reduces by half.

3. Strain into a large mug, using the back of a spoon to press as much liquid from the herbs as possible. Compost the solids.

4. Add the honey and allow the infusion to cool until it's comfortable to drink.

CONTINUED »

5. Swallow the borage oil capsule, either with a little cool water or with the tea. Have a small snack at the same time, as borage oil can cause indigestion when taken on an empty stomach. Drink the entire dose for best results. This remedy can be used daily if needed.

DEPRESSION

After-Shower Oil Spray

In depression, grooming is often one of the first things to be neglected. The herbs used in this oil spray have antibiotic and antibacterial properties and offer some deodorizing effects. Especially in cold weather or with older skin, a light spray of oil after the shower makes you feel more comfortable in your skin and keeps dry skin itchiness from gaining a foothold.

MAKES 3 OR 4 (½-CUP) APPLICATIONS

¼ cup alcohol-free witch hazel hydrosol

2 tablespoons sage-infused olive oil

2 tablespoons thyme-infused olive oil

2 tablespoons peppermint-infused olive oil

2 tablespoons lavender-infused olive oil

1. In a 1-cup glass measuring cup, combine the witch hazel and the sage-, thyme-, peppermint-, and lavender-infused olive oils.

2. Using a small funnel, transfer the oil mixture into a spray bottle. Label and date the bottle.

3. After a bath or shower, shake the contents well, then spray the oil mixture onto barely dry skin to soften and moisturize the body.

4. Massage the oil in well.

5. Store in a cool, dark place for up to 1 month.

Good Mood Blend

Essential oils, when diluted in a carrier oil such as fractionated coconut oil, can be massaged into the skin and then absorbed into the bloodstream. Diffusing the following essential oils can be effective in the treatment of depression.

MAKES 1 DOSE

2 drops clary sage
  essential oil

2 drops rose essential oil

2 drops basil
  essential oil

2 drops lavender
  essential oil

2 drops ylang-ylang
  essential oil

Place the clary sage, rose, basil, lavender, and ylang-ylang essential oils in a diffuser with the amount of water recommended in the manufacturer's instructions and inhale deeply. Use as desired.

Linden Syrup

It's great to have this syrup handy and ready to use in case someone in your household starts feeling low, ill, or restless. It can be taken by the tablespoon as medicine, or used to flavor tea, sparkling water, or food. While this recipe uses linden flowers and bracts and traditional honey, you can find linden honey made from the flowers to mix with the water and lemon instead. Like maple, the linden tree's sap can be gathered and boiled down to a syrup, which would also work mixed with water and lemon.

CONTINUED »

MAKES 2½ TO 3 CUPS

4 to 5 cups fresh linden
  flowers and bracts
1½ cups water
3 cups raw honey
Juice of 1 lemon

1. Clean the linden flowers and bracts by giving them a good shake and a quick dunk in water. Strain in a colander and set aside.

2. In a large pot, combine the water, honey, and lemon juice and simmer over low heat until thickened and reduced by about one-quarter.

3. Remove from the heat and add the flowers and bracts. Stir well and cover.

4. Let the syrup steep overnight, then strain into a bottle and compost the solids. Cap tightly, label, and date the bottle.

5. Store at room temperature and use within 1 year.

DEPRESSION

Spiced Licorice–Lemon Balm Infusion

Licorice, cloves, and lemon balm work together to lift feelings of minor depression. You can replace the lemon balm with peppermint, if you like. Omit the licorice root in this recipe if you have high blood pressure.

MAKES ABOUT 1 CUP

1 teaspoon dried
  chopped (cut and
  sifted) licorice root
1 tablespoon crushed
  dried lemon balm
3 whole cloves
1¼ cups water
Raw honey or stevia, for
  sweetening (optional)

1. In a small saucepan, combine the licorice, lemon balm, cloves, and water and bring to a boil over medium-high heat.

2. Reduce the heat to medium-low and simmer for 10 minutes.

3. Strain into a mug, using the back of a spoon to press the excess liquid from the herbs. Compost the solids.

CONTINUED »

4. Sweeten with honey (if using).

5. Enjoy a cup of this comforting tea anytime you need a mental lift.

DEPRESSION

St. John's Wort Infusion

St. John's wort is widely recognized as an excellent herbal remedy for mild depression. This infusion is suitable only for those who do not take prescription antidepressants, as it can cause an adverse reaction.

MAKES 1 DOSE

2 teaspoons dried St. John's wort flowers
½ teaspoon ground cinnamon
2 cups water
Raw honey or stevia, for sweetening

1. In a medium saucepan, combine the St. John's wort, cinnamon, and water and bring the mixture to a boil over medium-high heat.

2. Reduce the heat to medium-low and allow the infusion to simmer for 10 to 15 minutes, or until the liquid reduces by half.

3. Strain into a large mug, using the back of a spoon to press as much liquid from the herbs as possible. Compost the solids.

4. Add the honey and allow the infusion to cool until it's comfortable to drink.

5. Drink 3 cups a day, alongside a meal or snack to prevent nausea.

Uplifting St. John's Wort Smelling Salt

St. John's wort, lavender, and rosemary combine to ease feelings of mild depression. This smelling salt can be used alongside other treatments.

MAKES 1 OUNCE

1 ounce coarse sea salt

10 drops lavender essential oil

10 drops rosemary essential oil

10 drops St. John's wort essential oil

1. In a small, labeled jar, combine the salt and the lavender, rosemary, and St. John's wort essential oils.

2. Cap tightly and shake well to blend.

3. Inhale deeply for 20 seconds. Store in a cool, dark place for up to 1 year.

4. Use this remedy as often as you like. Refresh the blend with additional essential oil when the fragrance begins to fade.

Uplifting Tea

Certain herbs, such as St. John's wort, can boost your mood. Another example is eleuthero, which has been used in Eastern countries for centuries to help decrease cortisol levels and reduce depression. It is used to restore the balance of qi and improve vigor by stimulating a healthy appetite and enhancing overall health. Try making a daily ritual of sipping this herb-infused tea. The simple act of preparing and slowly sipping warm tea can also be therapeutic.

CONTINUED »

MAKES 4 CUPS

1 tablespoon dried St.
John's wort flowers

1 tablespoon dried
lemon balm

1 tablespoon dried, cut,
and sifted oatstraw

½ tablespoon dried
chamomile flowers

1. Place the St. John's wort, lemon balm, oatstraw, and chamomile in a French press, then fill the press with hot water.

2. Steep the mixture for 10 to 15 minutes, or up to 3 hours for a stronger infusion.

3. Pour the tea into a cup and drink. Compost the solids.

4. Store leftover tea in the refrigerator, labeled and dated, for up to 3 days.

EXHAUSTION AND FATIGUE

Awake and Aware Potion

This syrup contains herbs that relieve stress and the effects of it on the body and mind. At the same time, these herbs increase productivity. Yerba maté contains caffeine, and it provides many possible additional benefits. It's high in antioxidants, increases metabolism, and provides focus. Individuals taking MAOI medications should avoid yerba maté, as well as those with caffeine sensitivity.

**MAKES 32 SERVINGS
(16 OUNCES)**

2 cups water

2 tablespoons
schisandra berries

2 tablespoons
chopped dried
reishi mushrooms

2 tablespoons
eleuthero powder

2 tablespoons astragalus
root powder

1 cup raw honey

1 teaspoon yerba maté
tea leaves, or 1 tea bag
per 1 cup of potion

1. In a medium saucepan, combine the water, schisandra berries, reishi, eleuthero, and astragalus and bring to a boil over medium heat.

CONTINUED »

2. Reduce the heat to medium-low and simmer until the liquid reduces by half.

3. Strain into 2-cup glass measuring cup. It's okay if the liquid isn't quite 1 cup.

4. Put the honey in a medium bowl, then add the warm liquid and blend well.

5. Pour into 2 (8-ounce) jars, label, and date.

6. Brew a cup of yerba maté tea. Add 1 tablespoon of the honey syrup to the hot tea. (Remember, half of the syrup is herbal decoction, so it's just 1½ teaspoons honey.)

7. This syrup can be stored at room temperature for up to 1 week or in the refrigerator for up to 1 year.

EXHAUSTION AND FATIGUE

Energizing Ginseng Decoction

Whether you are physically exhausted or emotionally fatigued, you'll find that this energizing ginseng decoction serves as a wonderful pick-me-up. If you are often exhausted and have no explanation for frequent, overwhelming feelings of tiredness, see your doctor, as many illnesses, including some serious ones, are accompanied by symptoms of severe exhaustion and fatigue.

CONTINUED »

MAKES 1 DOSE

2 cups water

5 thin slices fresh
   ginseng root, or
   1½ teaspoons dried
   chopped (cut and
   sifted) ginseng root

1½ teaspoons grated
   fresh ginger

Raw honey or stevia,
   for sweetening

1. In a medium saucepan, combine the water, ginseng root, and ginger and bring the mixture to a boil over medium heat.

2. Reduce the heat to medium-low and allow the decoction to simmer for 10 to 15 minutes, or until the liquid reduces by half.

3. Remove the pan from the heat, cover it with a lid, and allow the decoction to rest for about 15 minutes.

4. Strain into a large mug, using the back of a spoon to press as much liquid from the herbs as possible. Compost the solids.

5. Add the honey before drinking.

6. Drink 1 dose a day.

EXHAUSTION AND FATIGUE

Giddyup Tea

Inertia is real! Having no energy leads to sitting (or lying) around, and that, in itself, takes away motivation. Feeling down or depressed can exacerbate this state of mind. This tea can help shift that mood and encourage energizing movement. Omit the licorice if you have high blood pressure.

MAKES 45 (1-CUP) SERVINGS

¼ cup green tea leaves

¼ cup dried chopped
   (cut and sifted)
   shatavari root

2 tablespoons dried
   holy basil

2 tablespoons dried
   chopped (cut and
   sifted) eleuthero root

1½ tablespoons dried
   schisandra berries

1½ tablespoons dried
   ginkgo leaf

1 tablespoon dried
   chopped (cut and
   sifted) licorice root

CONTINUED »

1. In a small bowl, combine the green tea, shatavari root, holy basil, eleuthero root, schisandra berries, ginkgo, and licorice root and mix well.

2. Place in a 1-cup container, label, and date.

3. Put 1 to 2 teaspoons of the blend in an infuser. Put the infuser in a 10-ounce mug and fill the mug with hot water. Steep for 10 minutes. Remove the infuser. Compost the solids. You can drink this tea daily.

4. Store the loose tea in a cool, dry place out of direct sunlight for up to 1 year.

EXHAUSTION AND FATIGUE

Motivational Chocolate

Cacao is considered a superfood, with a huge amount of antioxidants, magnesium, and other vitamins and minerals. Historically, maca has been used to increase strength, energy, stamina, and may even improve brain function when incorporated into the diet or daily herbal intake.

MAKES 8 SERVINGS

8 cups oat milk
1 cup raw cacao powder
¼ cup molasses
2 tablespoons maca powder
½ teaspoon cayenne pepper
⅛ teaspoon ground cardamom

1. Put the milk, cacao, molasses, maca, cayenne, and cardamom into a blender and blend on high speed for about a minute, or until the ingredients are smooth and well combined. (You can also premix the dry ingredients, then make smaller batches [e.g., ¼ cup of the premixed dry ingredients, 2 cups of oat milk, and 1 tablespoon of molasses] as needed.)

2. Pour the mixture into a medium saucepan, and warm over medium heat until the liquid

CONTINUED »

just reaches a simmer—warm enough to be "hot chocolate."

3. Label and date any leftover prepared drink. Store in the refrigerator and drink within 3 days.

4. If you premix the dry ingredients, store them in a cool, dry place in a labeled, dated, airtight container for up to 1 year.

EXHAUSTION AND FATIGUE

New Skin Sugar Scrub

Sugar scrubs do more than just make your skin look good and get rid of dry, scaly patches. The action of scrubbing wakes up the skin and gets blood circulation going. If you're feeling down and uncomfortable, clean, smooth skin goes a long way to making you feel better.

MAKES 2½ CUPS

1 cup sugar
½ cup grated soap
20 drops frankincense (boswellia) essential oil
20 drops orange essential oil
1 cup apricot kernel oil, almond oil, or sesame oil, plus more as needed

1. In a medium bowl, mix together the sugar, soap, frankincense oil, and orange oil.

2. Distribute the mixture evenly in wide-mouth plastic jars. I recommend using plastic jars because the oil on your hands can be slippery, and glass can break.

3. Divide the apricot kernel oil among the jars. A little more might be needed to cover the mixture with oil.

4. Label and date the jars and cover the labels with tape to protect them. Use within 1 year.

5. Standing in the tub or shower, scoop out a little of the mixture, and using your dry hands, begin with

CONTINUED »

scrubbing the feet, and work up the legs, including the buttocks. Then, begin at the hands and work toward the shoulders.

6. Rinse well and pat dry. Be very cautious of slipping in the tub or shower. Dry feet completely.

GRIEF

Grief Support Roller Bottle

Essential oils can stimulate chemical changes in brain chemistry by opening different neural pathways. Add essential oils to a roller bottle and massage over the chest. You can also add some essential oils to a bath and let the tears flow. Crying helps provide emotional release.

MAKES ⅓ OUNCE (1 ROLLER BOTTLE)

2 to 5 of the following essential oils:
Cedarwood essential oil
Frankincense (boswellia) essential oil
Rose essential oil
Clary sage essential oil
Geranium essential oil
Ginger essential oil
Lavender essential oil
Lemon balm essential oil
Jasmine essential oil
Neroli essential oil
Petitgrain essential oil
10 milliliters fractionated coconut oil

1. Put 2 drops each of the essential oils you have chosen in a 10-milliliter roller bottle.

2. Fill the bottle to the top with fractionated coconut oil.

3. Massage in a circular motion over the heart and lungs.

4. Use as needed. Store in a cool, dry place and use within 1 year.

Healing Heart Tonic

Grieving is a natural process almost everyone must endure at some time. While healing from the loss of a loved one, this fragrant tonic brings a restorative sense of calm and peace, promotes emotional transcendence, and helps your mind relax. It is also useful for easing anxiety and mild depression.

MAKES 1 DOSE

4 cups water

2 tablespoons dried hibiscus flower

2 tablespoons dried rose petals

2 tablespoons dried hawthorn berries

2 tablespoons dried lavender flowers

Raw honey or stevia, for sweetening

1 drop rose essential oil diluted in 1 teaspoon sweet almond oil

1. In a medium saucepan, combine the water, hibiscus, rose petals, hawthorn berries, and lavender flowers and bring the mixture to a boil over medium-high heat.

2. Reduce the heat and allow the tonic to simmer for 10 to 15 minutes, or until the liquid reduces by half.

3. Strain into a large mug, using the back of a spoon to press as much liquid from the herbs as possible. Add the honey before drinking. Compost the solids.

4. Dab essential oil on each temple, inhaling deeply as you consume the tonic. Drink the entire dose. Repeat as needed, drinking up to 3 cups a day.

Foundational Focus Elixir

This combination is specifically helpful for those periods of time when you have to perform at high levels for a stretch of time. Things like cramming for finals, writing a term paper, the last month before the house sale finally goes

CONTINUED »

through, or filing taxes are examples that come to mind. It can also be useful on vacation, because even though trips are something we've looked forward to all year, we push our bodies and take in so much information that a little focus can help a lot.

MAKES ABOUT 3 OUNCES

2 tablespoons dried chopped (cut and sifted) ashwagandha root

2 tablespoons dried chopped (cut and sifted) rhodiola root

2 tablespoons dried chopped (cut and sifted) eleuthero root

2 tablespoons raw honey

Vodka to cover (a little more than 4 tablespoons)

1. In a small (4-ounce) jar, combine the ashwagandha, rhodiola, and eleuthero.

2. Add the honey. Using a knife or chopstick, combine the honey with the herbs.

3. Fill the rest of the jar with the vodka. Put a lid on the jar and shake well.

4. Infuse the elixir for 2 to 4 weeks, storing it in a cool, dark place and shaking occasionally.

5. Once it's done infusing, strain the elixir and transfer it to a dropper bottle. Compost the solids.

6. Label and date the elixir.

7. Take up to 1 teaspoon of elixir 2 times a day.

8. Store the elixir in a cool, dark place for up to 3 years.

LACK OF FOCUS

No Excuses Tincture

This is a terrific synergistic combination of herbs for calm, focused energy. The list of benefits goes on and on, and includes relief from stress and improved memory, but we've got the adaptogens and they help balance everything out. This is truly an impressive blend.

CONTINUED »

MAKES 1 PINT

¼ cup dried chopped
  (cut and sifted)
  rhodiola root
¼ cup dried chopped
  (cut and sifted)
  ashwagandha root
¼ cup dried chopped
  (cut and sifted)
  shatavari root
¼ cup dried chopped
  (cut and sifted)
  eleuthero root
2¼ cups vodka

1. In a quart jar, combine the rhodiola root, ashwa-gandha root, shatavari root, eleuthero root, and vodka. Mix very well to get rid of clumps. Cover with a lid.

2. Allow to infuse for 4 weeks, giving the jar a good shake every day if you can remember. It helps to have it on the counter (away from heat and direct sunlight) where it's noticed daily.

3. After a month, strain into a bottle and compost the solids. Label with the date, ingredients, and instructions for use.

4. Take 40 drops 1 to 2 times a day.

5. Store in a cool place out of direct sunlight. It will last indefinitely.

LACK OF MENTAL CLARITY

Clear Thoughts Tea Blend

All the herbs and roots combined in this delicious tea work together to awaken and energize your mind. It can put a little spring in your step, too. Make this in two parts because the roots require a different extraction method than the herbal infusion.

MAKES 30 (1-CUP) SERVINGS

For the syrup

1 tablespoon grated
  fresh ginger

1 tablespoon dried
  chopped (cut and
  sifted) rhodiola root
¾ cup water
⅓ cup raw honey

For the tea blend and
the infusion

¼ cup dried rosemary
¼ cup dried chopped
  (cut and sifted)
  astragalus root
¼ cup dried peppermint

CONTINUED »

1. In a small saucepan, combine the ginger, rhodiola, and water and bring to a boil over medium-high heat.

2. Reduce the heat to medium-low and simmer the mixture until the liquid reduces by half.

3. Strain into a bowl and compost the solids.

4. Add the honey to the strained liquid and mix well to combine.

5. Transfer the syrup to a bottle. Label and date the syrup.

6. Refrigerate the syrup for up to 3 months.

To make the tea blend and infusion

7. In a large bowl, combine the rosemary, astragalus, and peppermint.

8. Transfer the tea blend to an airtight container. Label and date the blend.

9. To use, put 1 rounded teaspoon of the blend in an infuser and place it in a 10-ounce mug. Cover with boiling water and let steep for 5 minutes. Remove the infuser. Compost the solids.

10. Add 2 teaspoons of the ginger-rhodiola syrup.

11. Store the loose tea in a cool, dry place out of direct sunlight for up to 1 year.

Good Memory Elixir

Herbs for stimulating circulation in every part of the brain, protecting the capillaries, and helping with balancing moods swim in the sweetened brandy and become just the thing for clearing a groggy head. Using this elixir in conjunction with anticoagulants could make the blood too thin. Consult with your doctor before using if you are on blood medication.

MAKES ABOUT 2 CUPS

¼ **cup dried ginkgo leaves**

¼ **cup dried gotu kola**

¼ **cup dried chopped (cut and sifted) eleuthero root**

¼ **cup dried hawthorn berries**

1 **tablespoon grated fresh ginger**

½ **cup molasses**

2 **cups brandy**

1. In a quart jar, combine the ginkgo, gotu kola, eleuthero root, hawthorn berries, ginger, molasses, and brandy; mix well to remove any air pockets and dissolve the molasses in the brandy.

2. Let the mixture infuse for 3 to 4 weeks.

3. Strain into a bottle and compost the solids. Label with the date, ingredients, and instructions for use.

4. Take 1 teaspoon of the elixir once or twice a day.

5. Store in a cool place out of direct sunlight for up to 1 year.

Pine Needle Tea

Be sure to make this tea with fresh or frozen-from-fresh pine needles. Dried needles lose their vibrancy very quickly. The flavor of the tea is not as strong as you might think. Some people love the flavor as is, but I like to add something else like hibiscus, peppermint, or lemon—and always honey!

CONTINUED »

MAKES 2 CUPS

2¼ cups water
½ cup fresh pine
needles, cleaned and
cut into ½-inch pieces
Raw honey, for
sweetening (optional)

1. In a small saucepan, bring the water to a boil over medium-high heat.

2. Add the pine needles to the boiling water, then remove the pan from the heat.

3. Cover and let steep for 3 to 5 minutes.

4. Strain and compost the solids. Allow to cool slightly before sweetening with honey (if using) and drinking.

LACK OF MENTAL CLARITY

Rosemary-Citrus Temple Rub

Natural emollients and energizing essential oils come together in this invigorating rub that will help clear brain fog.

MAKES 20 DOSES

1 tablespoon olive oil
1 tablespoon jojoba oil
1½ teaspoons finely
grated beeswax
15 drops rosemary
essential oil
15 drops tangerine
essential oil

1. In a medium saucepan, warm the olive oil, jojoba oil, and beeswax over low to medium-low heat just until the beeswax melts. Mix thoroughly and remove the saucepan from the heat. Stir in the rosemary and tangerine essential oils.

2. Pour the mixture into a small wide-mouth container. Allow the mixture to cool completely before capping. Label and date the container.

3. Apply 1 to 2 drops to your forehead or temples when you need a lift. Feel free to use the rub as a deeply penetrating moisturizer for dry skin on hands, feet, elbows, and other areas as needed.

4. Keep in a cool, dark place for up to 1 year.

Tonic Granola Bars with Holy Basil, Astragalus, and Ashwagandha

These granola bars are a great way to start the day and wake up your brain. An easy, grab-and-go breakfast when you're on the run—they're delicious and provide a terrific boost. No baking required!

MAKES 8 TO 10 BARS

4 tablespoons (½ stick) butter, plus more for greasing

2 cups quick oats

1 cup crispy rice cereal

¼ cup peanuts

¼ cup pumpkin seeds or pistachios

¼ cup mini chocolate chips

1 tablespoon holy basil powder

1 tablespoon astragalus root powder

1 tablespoon ashwagandha root powder

1 tablespoon minced crystallized ginger

¼ teaspoon salt

¼ cup packed brown sugar

¼ cup raw honey

½ cup peanut butter

1 teaspoon vanilla extract

1. Grease a 9-by-9-inch baking pan with butter.

2. In a large bowl, stir together the oats, cereal, peanuts, pumpkin seeds, chocolate chips, holy basil, astragalus, ashwagandha, ginger, and salt. Set aside.

3. In a large saucepan, bring the butter, brown sugar, honey, and peanut butter to a low boil over medium-low heat for 3 to 4 minutes. Remove from the heat and stir in the vanilla, followed by the dry ingredients. Mix well.

4. Spread the mixture evenly in the prepared baking pan and refrigerate for 1 hour before cutting and serving.

5. The granola bars can be stored in a labeled, dated, airtight container in the refrigerator for up to 10 days.

Up in Smoke Incense

This is a wonderful little ritual to try when it is impossible to move on because it feels like nothing is working and there are too many things blocking the way—real or imagined.

MAKES 1 TABLESPOON

1 teaspoon crushed
   dried sage
1 teaspoon powdered
   dragon's blood or
   frankincense resin
1 teaspoon
   ground cinnamon

1. In a small jar, blend together the sage, dragon's blood, and cinnamon. Label with the ingredients, date, and instructions for use.

2. Outdoors, light an incense charcoal block and place it in a heatproof incense burner.

3. While it is heating, write the problems or blockages you're experiencing on small pieces of paper. You can write longer descriptions or single words, like names or places.

4. Sprinkle a pinch of the incense blend on the charcoal. As it smokes, ball up the paper and put that on the charcoal, one piece at a time.

5. Add more incense if there are lots of pieces of paper.

6. Sit back and watch your troubles float away.

7. Store the jar in a cool, dark place. It will last indefinitely.

Basil-Citrus Aromatherapy Treatment

Lift your spirits and boost emotions by diffusing an invigorating blend of essential oils in your home or office. If you don't have a diffuser, you can dab a few drops of this essential oil blend onto a lamp's lightbulb while cool, turn on the lamp, and enjoy the energizing, uplifting fragrances anywhere you happen to be.

MAKES 5 TO 25 DOSES

20 drops basil
  essential oil

20 drops lemon
  essential oil

40 drops grapefruit
  essential oil

20 drops peppermint
  essential oil

1. In a dark-colored glass bottle with a narrow neck, combine the basil, lemon, grapefruit, and peppermint essential oils. Label and date the bottle; this treatment will keep for up to 2 years.

2. Add the mixture, 15 to 20 drops at a time, to a diffuser with the amount of water recommended in the manufacturer's instructions and inhale deeply. Alternatively, use up to 5 drops at a time on standard lightbulbs, adding before the light is turned on.

Coffee Sugar Scrub

Coffee scrubs are so good at increasing blood flow and making facial skin look alive and glowing that they actually boost the mood. It doesn't hurt that they also smell wonderful. They exfoliate while the antiaging caffeine hydrates.

CONTINUED »

MAKES 1 CUP

⅓ cup fresh finely
   ground coffee
¼ cup jojoba oil
⅓ cup packed
   brown sugar
1 tablespoon melted
   cocoa butter

1. In a small bowl, combine the coffee, jojoba oil, sugar, and cocoa butter and mix well.

2. Divide into 2 or 3 wide-mouth plastic jars. Label and date the sugar scrub.

3. This can be used on the body as well as the face. Avoid the eye area and sensitive skin areas on the body.

4. Some people prefer to use soap first and just rinse off the scrub, some like to wash after. Either way, leave the scrub on the skin for several minutes.

5. Keep the jar closed between uses. Sugar scrubs are stable as long as there is no water introduced into the mix.

LOW MOOD

Daily Mood Support Honey

This honey can be used to sweeten any tea, morning oatmeal, or cereal or enjoyed by the teaspoon. Add a bit to some vinegar and use it as a salad dressing. There are lots of ways to get a little daily mood support.

MAKES ABOUT 1 CUP

2 tablespoons
   dried chopped
   (cut and sifted)
   ashwagandha root
2 tablespoons dried
   holy basil

2 tablespoons dried
   chopped (cut and
   sifted) rhodiola root

2 tablespoons
   dried chopped
   (cut and sifted)
   eleuthero root
1 cup raw honey

CONTINUED »

1. In a pint jar, combine the ashwagandha, holy basil, rhodiola, eleuthero, and honey.

2. Mix well, making sure to remove all the air bubbles.

3. Seal the jar, and label and date the blend.

4. Infuse the honey for 3 to 4 weeks, storing it in a cool, dark place. The herbs will migrate to the top of the honey, so turn the jar over each day.

5. Strain into a jar for a few hours to get as much of the honey as possible. Compost the solids. Label and date the blend.

6. Honey is very stable at room temperature, especially when stored in a cool, dark place. It will last at least 1 year. If you wish, you can also store it in the refrigerator for the same amount of time.

LOW MOOD

Happy Day Room Spray

A spray can change the whole feel of a space. When a room starts to feel heavy and stagnant, it's time for a quick change. Choosing light citrus essential oils will lift the spirits. Think about how you feel when someone near you tears the skin off an orange. The basil essential oil can improve mood and alertness as well.

MAKES 8 OUNCES

¾ **cup water**

¼ **cup vodka**

30 drops lemon essential oil

30 drops grapefruit essential oil

15 drops basil essential oil

CONTINUED »

1. In an 8-ounce spray bottle, combine the water, vodka, lemon essential oil, grapefruit essential oil, and basil essential oil. Label and date the spray.

2. Spray a few spritzes into the air anytime you need a shift in energy or to lighten the mood in the room.

3. Store the spray in a cool, dark place for up to 1 year.

MEMORY ISSUES

Diffused Rosemary

Rosemary essential oil may be able to boost memory. All you have to do is breathe it in, especially if you are doing a task that requires focus.

MAKES 1 DOSE

4 to 5 drops rosemary essential oil

Place the essential oils in a diffuser with the amount of water recommended in the manufacturer's instructions and inhale deeply.

MEMORY ISSUES

Ginger-Ginkgo Decoction

Both ginger and ginkgo enhance blood flow, energizing the mind and stimulating the memory.

MAKES 2 TO 4 DOSES

8 cups water

16 thin slices dried ginkgo root

4 tablespoons grated fresh ginger

Raw honey or stevia, for sweetening

CONTINUED »

1. In a large pot, combine the water, ginkgo root, and ginger and bring the mixture to a boil over medium-high heat.

2. Reduce the heat to medium-low and allow the decoction to simmer for 10 to 15 minutes, or until the liquid reduces by half.

3. Remove the pot from the heat, cover it with a lid, and allow the decoction to rest for about 15 minutes.

4. Strain the decoction into a jar, using the back of a spoon to press as much liquid from the herbs as possible. Compost the solids. Add honey to taste, then label and date the jar.

5. Drink 1 to 2 cups per day, hot or over ice.

6. Store, covered, in the refrigerator for up to 1 week.

MEMORY ISSUES

Green Tea with Ginseng and Sage

Green tea, ginseng, and sage combine to boost the chemicals responsible for transmitting messages within your brain.

MAKES 1 CUP

1 tablespoon crushed dried sage

1 teaspoon dried chopped (cut and sifted) ginseng root

1 cup boiling water

1 green tea bag

Raw honey or stevia, for sweetening (optional)

Freshly squeezed lemon juice, for serving (optional)

CONTINUED »

1. Place the sage and ginseng in a tea ball or infuser. Fill a mug with the boiling water, then add the tea ball and the green tea bag.

2. Steep for 15 minutes. Remove the tea ball and the tea bag. Compost the solids.

3. Sweeten with honey (if using). Add lemon juice if the sage flavor seems too strong.

4. Enjoy 2 to 3 cups of this tea each day during the morning and early afternoon hours.

MEMORY ISSUES

Remember More Tea

There are herbs that are known to increase circulation in the small capillaries in the brain. Others protect the brain, and others stimulate the brain. There is a gold mine of these herbs in this tea. And it tastes pretty good, too! This tea used in conjunction with anticoagulants could make the blood too thin. Discuss with your doctor before using if on you are on blood medication.

MAKES 96 (1-CUP) SERVINGS
½ **cup dried ginkgo leaf**
½ **cup dried gotu kola**
¼ **cup dried hibiscus**
¼ **cup dried chopped (cut and sifted) eleuthero root**
¼ **cup dried bacopa**
2 **tablespoons dried rosemary**
1 **tablespoon ground ginger**

1. In a medium bowl, combine the ginkgo, gotu kola, hibiscus, eleuthero root, bacopa, rosemary, and ginger.

2. Transfer to a pint container. Label with the ingredients, date, and name.

3. Put 1 or 2 teaspoons of the blend in an infuser. Put the infuser in a 10-ounce mug and fill the mug with boiling water. Steep for 5 minutes. Remove the infuser. Compost the solids.

CONTINUED »

4. Drink 1 to 3 cups a day.

5. Store the loose tea in a cool, dry place out of direct sunlight for up to 1 year.

MEMORY ISSUES

Rosemary Smelling Salt

Rosemary essential oil helps improve memory, reduce anxiety, and promote an overall sense of well-being. Use this treatment alone or in combination with others.

MAKES 1 OUNCE

1 ounce coarse sea salt
20 drops rosemary essential oil

1. In a small glass jar, combine the sea salt and the rosemary essential oil.

2. Cover and shake well to blend.

3. Breathe deeply for 20 seconds. Store in a cool, dark place for up to 1 year.

4. Use this remedy regularly, particularly when undertaking cognitive tasks. If you like, you can leave the jar open near your work area. Refresh the smelling salt with more essential oil when the fragrance begins to fade.

NERVOUSNESS

Let It Go Toddy

Particularly nice on a cold winter night, this twist on a classic comforting drink is very flexible and can be easily altered by making an infusion with the hot water, using infused honey, or completely swapping out the herbs. This recipe is meant to be shared. If only one person will be drinking it, halve the recipe.

CONTINUED »

MAKES 2 SERVINGS

1½ cups hot water

1 tablespoon raw honey

2 tablespoons lavender-
   infused vinegar

1 tablespoon
   hawthorn tincture

1 tablespoon lemon
   balm tincture

2 lemon wedges

1. In a 2-cup glass measuring cup, combine the water, honey, and vinegar. Mix well to combine.

2. Stir in the hawthorn and lemon balm tinctures.

3. Divide the mixture into two teacups.

4. Garnish with a wedge of lemon and enjoy warm.

NERVOUSNESS

Nerve Support Elixir

This elixir combines herbs that address more acute nervous upsets and go on to support and nourish nerves to increase resilience. Measurements of the honey and alcohol will vary depending on the size of jar you use. Use the ingredients list as a rough guideline.

MAKES 6 OUNCES

2 tablespoons
   dried skullcap

2 tablespoons
   dried motherwort

2 tablespoons dried
   chamomile flowers

2 tablespoons dried
   chopped (cut and
   sifted) astragalus root

2 tablespoons
   milky oats

⅓ cup raw honey

½ cup alcohol (vodka,
   rum, or any
   alcohol of choice)

1. In a medium (at least 8-ounce) jar, combine the skullcap, motherwort, chamomile, astragalus, and milky oats.

2. Add the honey until the jar is about one-third full, using a knife to mix it with the herbs.

3. Fill the rest of the jar with your alcohol of choice. Cover the jar and shake well.

CONTINUED »

4. Infuse the elixir for 2 to 4 weeks, storing it in a cool, dark place and shaking occasionally.

5. Once it's done infusing, strain the elixir and transfer it to a 6-ounce dropper bottle. Compost the solids.

6. Label and date the elixir.

7. Take 1 dropperful (25 drops) each morning and/or evening as needed.

8. Store the elixir in a cool, dark place for up to 3 years.

RESTLESSNESS

Perchance to Dream Pillow

When my sister and I were herb ladies at a Renaissance festival, we made dream pillows to help with sleep. We heard over and over that people would wake, hold the pillow against their face, and drop back to sleep. I've learned of tales of workers in hops fields falling asleep while they labor, and I'm certain lavender fields are responsible for their fair share of nappers, too. Some people have very vivid dreams with mugwort. Discontinue use if it causes a problem.

MAKES 1 PILLOW

¼ **cup dried hops**

¼ **cup dried lavender flowers**

¼ **cup dried chamomile flowers**

¼ **cup dried catnip**

¼ **cup dried mugwort**

1. Sew together 3 sides of 2 (6-inch) squares of fabric, with the outward-facing sides together.

2. Turn the fabric pouch inside out and fill it with the hops, lavender, chamomile, catnip, and mugwort.

3. Turn in the edges of the open end and sew them shut.

CONTINUED »

4. When needed, place this packet inside the pillow-case of a regular bed pillow, and store in a plastic bag in a cool, dry place between uses.

5. Do not wash the herb-filled packet; if it gets wet, the herbs will not dry properly and will likely grow moldy. Replace when the scent has faded, within 1 to 5 years, depending on how often it is used.

RESTLESSNESS

Sweet Dreams Elixir

At one time, if a person was visibly shaken by events, it was completely normal to offer them a small amount of alcohol, often brandy, in a truly medicinal way. Though not everyone wants to or can consume alcohol, for those who do, this can have a calming effect. Add some herbs, and it takes on a whole different aspect.

MAKES ABOUT 10 OUNCES

1 cup fresh
   chamomile flowers
1 cup fresh lemon balm
1 tablespoon grated
   fresh ginger
¼ cup raw honey
1½ cups brandy, or
   enough to cover all
   the herbs

1. In a 1-quart jar, combine the chamomile, lemon balm, and ginger.

2. Add the honey and stir well to coat everything. Add the brandy.

3. Allow everything to steep together for 2 to 4 weeks.

4. Strain into a bottle and compost the solids. Label with the date, ingredients, and instructions for use. An ounce or two is enough to settle the mind and let a peaceful night fall.

5. Store the elixir in a cool, dark place for up to 3 years.

Rose and Raspberry Jam

In this jam, the flavor and scent of the roses combine with the raspberries in an almost magical way. Plus, the raspberries contain pectin, so the fruit sets up on its own. The deep, dark berries add antioxidants to all the great benefits of the roses. Spread this jam on your English muffin in the morning to start your day off right.

MAKES 3½ CUPS

1½ cups water
2 cups fresh rose petals
1 cup fresh
    black raspberries
2 cups sugar
1 tablespoon freshly
    squeezed lemon juice

1. Place the water and rose petals in a food processor and pulse to chop the petals into smaller pieces.

2. Pour the mixture into a medium saucepan and add the berries. Bring to a boil over high heat, then reduce the heat to low and simmer for 10 minutes.

3. Add the sugar and lemon juice, stirring to dissolve the sugar.

4. Simmer for another 20 to 30 minutes.

5. Remove from the heat and pour into hot sterilized jars. When they cool, label and date the jars.

6. Store the jam in the refrigerator for 2 to 3 months.

Liquid Sunshine Tincture

There is no such thing as liquid sunshine, but if there were, it would likely look something like this bottle of herbal cheer. St. John's wort got its name because it blooms around the summer solstice, which coincides with the Feast of St. John on June 24. To celebrate the longest day of light, the blossoms were

CONTINUED »

gathered and used to create head wreaths and bouquets. Bonfires were lit to represent the light.

MAKES 4 OUNCES

2 tablespoons St. John's wort tincture

2 tablespoons mimosa tincture

2 tablespoons lemon balm tincture

2 tablespoons rhodiola tincture

2 tablespoons water or juice (per dose)

1. In a 1-cup glass measuring cup, combine the St. John's wort, mimosa, lemon balm, and rhodiola tinctures.

2. Transfer the mixture into a 4-ounce dropper bottle.

3. Label and date the tincture blend.

4. Take 1 dropperful (25 drops) in the water or juice up to 3 times a day as needed.

5. Store the tincture blend in a cool, dark place for up to 3 years.

SEASONAL AFFECTIVE DISORDER (SAD)

Uplifting Citrus Body Balm

Natural moisturizers and uplifting essential oils come together in this delightful body balm, which boosts spirits and helps heal dry, winter-worn skin.

MAKES 30 DOSES

1 cup cocoa butter

½ cup avocado oil

½ cup jojoba oil

½ cup coconut oil

40 drops tangerine essential oil

10 drops chamomile essential oil

1. In a medium saucepan, combine the cocoa butter, avocado oil, jojoba oil, and coconut oil over low to medium-low heat, warming just until the coconut oil melts. Mix the ingredients thoroughly, then remove the pan from the heat.

2. Add the tangerine and chamomile essential oils and blend thoroughly.

3. Pour the mixture into a wide-mouth jar. Allow the balm to cool completely before capping. Label and date the jar.

CONTINUED »

4. To use, apply the balm to the skin after bathing or showering, and reapply it to the hands as needed.

5. Store the balm in a cool, dark place for up to 1 year.

SLEEP ISSUES

Go to Sleep Now Tincture

Sleep makes such a difference in how well we can manage in the world, but so often it's elusive when we need it the most. Sleep resets our brains and puts us back together. I love this tincture because it is a relaxing sedative and slows a racing brain to a crawl.

MAKES 4 OUNCES

4 tablespoons California poppy tincture

2 tablespoons passionflower tincture

2 tablespoons skullcap tincture

1. In a 1-cup glass measuring cup, combine the California poppy, passionflower, and skullcap tinctures.

2. Transfer the mixture to a 4-ounce dropper bottle. Label and date the tincture blend.

3. Take 1 to 2 dropperfuls (25 to 50 drops) on their own 30 minutes before bed.

4. Store the tincture blend in a cool, dark place for up to 3 years.

SLEEP ISSUES

Lavender-Chamomile Sleep Balm

Peaceful essential oils make this soothing sleep balm perfect for use when you're feeling restless but need to sleep.

CONTINUED »

MAKES 4 OUNCES

1 tablespoon olive oil

1 tablespoon jojoba oil

1½ teaspoons finely grated beeswax

15 drops lavender essential oil

15 drops chamomile essential oil

1. In a medium saucepan, combine the olive oil, jojoba oil, and beeswax over low to medium-low heat, warming just until the beeswax melts. Mix thoroughly and remove the saucepan from the heat.

2. Add the lavender and chamomile essential oils, blend thoroughly, and pour the mixture into a small wide-mouth container. Label and date the container, and allow the balm to cool completely before capping.

3. Apply the balm to your temples at bedtime, preferably after enjoying a warm bath or shower.

4. Store in a cool, dark place for up to 1 year.

SLEEP ISSUES

Monster Spray

Many years ago, we made gallons of this spray in our shop. Initially it was surprising to hear the parents tell us how it helped their children sleep better. Kids like being able to spray under the bed or in the closet before going to sleep, and the essential oils help them fall asleep. It works for grownups, too!

MAKES 1 SPRAY

¾ cup water

¼ cup vodka

30 drops tangerine essential oil

20 drops chamomile essential oil

10 drops lavender essential oil

1. In an 8-ounce spray bottle, combine the water, vodka, tangerine essential oil, chamomile essential oil, and lavender essential oil.

2. A fanciful label is fun to make for this concoction! Perhaps a coat of arms, a superhero, or the child could draw a picture of a monster.

3. Keep the spray on the child's nightstand for easy access, should a monster appear. It can be kept for up to 5 years.

Sleep Tight Formula

Have you ever had a night when you just can't seem to fall asleep? Tossing and turning, lightly drifting off, only to be woken by a noise or twitchy leg? This formula helps turn off chattery thoughts, relax you, and get you to fall asleep. If difficulty falling asleep is a common occurrence, consider altering your nighttime routine to include a relaxing Epsom salts bath and no electronic devices for at least an hour before bedtime. Regular exercise can also help improve sleep patterns.

MAKES 4 OUNCES

2 tablespoons
  chamomile tincture

2 tablespoons
  lavender tincture

2 tablespoons
  rose tincture

2 tablespoons
  passionflower tincture

1. In a 1-cup glass measuring cup, combine the chamomile tincture, lavender tincture, rose tincture, and passionflower tincture and mix well.

2. Pour the tincture blend into a 4-ounce glass dropper bottle. Tighten the dropper lid on the bottle and label with the name of the formula, the date, and the dosage information.

3. Add 1 to 2 dropperfuls (25 to 50 drops) tincture blend to a small glass of water or juice and drink before bed, repeating after 20 minutes if needed.

4. Store the bottle in a cool, dark place for up to 3 years.

Zonk Me Out Tea Blend

This is a real knockout blend of herbs. Enjoy in the evening to get a good night's sleep. Each of the herbs, when used alone, relaxes us in a slightly different way. Combining them allows us to relieve almost all the possible issues with sleep.

CONTINUED »

**MAKES 30 TO 35
(1-CUP) SERVINGS**

1 cup dried
  passionflower
¼ cup dried hops
¼ cup dried lemon balm
¼ cup dried
  chamomile flowers
1 tablespoon dried
  California poppy
1 tablespoon
  dried skullcap
Raw honey, for
  sweetening (optional)

1. In a pint jar, combine the passionflower, hops, lemon balm, chamomile, California poppy, and skullcap. Label and date the jar.

2. To use, make a strong infusion by putting 2 rounded teaspoons of loose tea in an infuser. Place the infuser in a 10-ounce mug. Cover with boiling water and steep for 10 to 15 minutes. Remove the infuser. Compost the solids.

3. Add honey (if using).

4. Store the loose tea in a cool, dark place for up to 1 year.

SOCIAL ANXIETY

Calm Balm

This soothing balm is particularly good to use before and during getting back out into public after extended periods of alone time. Or (as I can personally attest to) when it becomes necessary for an introvert to pretend to be an extrovert. It can be applied to hands, elbows, knees, temples, and anywhere the scent or skin-soothing properties would benefit. It's even a good lip balm.

MAKES ABOUT 4 OUNCES

⅜ cup coconut oil
1 (3-inch) vanilla
  bean, chopped
¼ cup dried
  lavender flowers

2 ounces cocoa butter
½ ounce beeswax

10 drops lavender
  essential oil (optional)

1. In an ovenproof bowl or ceramic dish, combine the coconut oil, vanilla bean, and lavender. Put the bowl in the oven at the lowest setting for 2 hours, then strain the mixture into a small heatproof bowl and compost the solids.

CONTINUED »

2. Add the cocoa butter and beeswax while the strained liquid is still warm. Either return to the oven to melt, or melt in the microwave in 30-second bursts until just liquid. If the lavender scent is too faint, stir in the lavender essential oil.

3. Pour into small jars, then label and date the balm. Allow the balm to harden before screwing on the lids.

4. Store in a cool, dark place for up to 1 year.

SOCIAL ANXIETY

Friendship Tea

Some people naturally experience social awkwardness and shyness. Lemon balm, passionflower, lavender, and ginkgo help calm nerves and elevate mood to support healthy social interaction. If you take any medications, be sure to talk with a health-care professional about potential interactions before using any of these herbs.

MAKES 32 DOSES

½ **cup chopped dried ginkgo**
½ **cup dried passionflower**
½ **cup dried lemon balm**
½ **cup dried peppermint**
1 **tablespoon dried lavender flowers**
1 **cup water (per dose)**
Raw honey or stevia, for sweetening (optional)

1. In a medium glass container, combine the ginkgo, passionflower, lemon balm, peppermint, and lavender. Seal, label, and date the tea blend. It will keep in a cool, dark place for up to 1 year.

2. To use, put 1 rounded teaspoon in an infuser and place it in a 10-ounce mug. Cover with boiling water and steep for 5 minutes. Remove the infuser, and sweeten the tea with honey (if using). Compost the solids.

3. Drink up to 3 cups a day.

Before-the-Storm Nerve Tonic Oxymel

An oxymel is very much like an elixir, but you replace the alcohol with apple cider vinegar. This blend combines adaptogens, which are herbs that specifically help your body adapt to and manage stress. It calms and supports the nervous system and can be used on a regular basis.

MAKES 16 OUNCES

2 tablespoons dried chopped (cut and sifted) ashwagandha root

2 tablespoons dried chopped (cut and sifted) astragalus root

2 tablespoons dried lemon balm

2 tablespoons dried chamomile flowers

2 tablespoons dried holy basil

2 tablespoons dried chopped (cut and sifted) eleuthero root

½ cup raw honey

2 cups apple cider vinegar

1 tablespoon to ½ cup water or juice (per dose)

1. In a 1-quart wide-mouth jar, combine the ashwagandha, astragalus, lemon balm, chamomile, holy basil, and eleuthero.

2. Add the honey and stir with a long spoon to combine with the herbs.

3. Add the vinegar and mix well.

4. Cover with a plastic lid or top the jar with a square of parchment paper before covering with a metal lid to prevent it from rusting.

5. Infuse the oxymel for 2 to 4 weeks, storing it in a cool, dark place and shaking occasionally.

6. Once it's done infusing, strain into a bottle and compost the solids. Label and date the oxymel.

7. Add 1 tablespoon oxymel to water or juice and drink daily.

8. Store in a cool, dry place out of direct sunlight for up to 1 year.

Cup of Kindness

Orange blossom water works hard to fight anxiety and stress, and tastes great doing it! Holy basil is one of the top adaptogens to help fight stress. This tea is delightful hot or iced.

Orange blossom water, like rose water, is a hydrosol, steam-distilled from the blossoms of oranges.

MAKES 1 SERVING

1 teaspoon dried
  holy basil
1 cup hot water
1 teaspoon orange
  blossom water
1 teaspoon raw honey
Orange wedge or twist,
  for serving (optional)

1. Steep the holy basil in the hot water for 5 minutes. Strain and add the orange blossom water and honey. Compost the solids.

2. A cup of this beverage seems too good to be good for you! With the addition of a wedge of orange, it feels downright decadent.

Herbal Almond Bliss Balls

These delicious morsels include plenty of anti-stress and energizing properties hidden in the form of a treat. I sometimes think this is the kind of thing that is best shared with the people stressing you out. There are plenty in this recipe to pass around.

MAKES ABOUT 50 BALLS

For the bliss balls

1 cup almond butter

2 tablespoons
  coconut oil
½ cup shredded coconut

½ cup chopped dates
½ cup raw honey

CONTINUED »

¼ cup ashwagandha
    root powder
¼ cup astragalus
    root powder
¼ cup eleuthero powder
1 tablespoon
    ground ginger
1 teaspoon salt

For the coating blend

¼ cup finely
    chopped almonds
¼ cup shredded coconut
¼ cup cocoa powder

To make the bliss balls

1. In a medium bowl, combine the almond butter, coconut oil, shredded coconut, dates, and honey and blend well.

2. In a small bowl, combine the ashwagandha, astragalus, eleuthero, ginger, and salt, and blend well.

3. Pour the powder mixture into the bowl with the almond butter mixture and stir well until everything is fully incorporated.

4. Cover and chill dough in the refrigerator for 30 minutes.

To coat the bliss balls

5. In a small bowl, make the coating blend by combining the almonds, coconut, and cocoa powder.

6. Shape the dough into 1- to 1½-inch balls. Roll in the coating mixture, pressing it into the ball, and cover the surface.

7. Eat 1 or 2 balls a day.

8. Store in a labeled, dated, airtight container in the refrigerator for 2 to 3 weeks or in the freezer for up to 3 months.

STRESS

Lavender Sachet

These simple sacks of herbs come in handy in innumerable ways. You can tuck them into drawers or closets, into your car to keep it smelling pleasant, in the

CONTINUED »

bedside table to reach for during a restless night, or in a desk drawer or locker to pull out on bad days at work or school. Unless exposed to bright light and heat, dried lavender retains its scent indefinitely. If the scent fades, scrunch the sachet a few times to refresh it.

MAKES 1 SACHET

1 cup dried
  lavender buds

Pour the dried lavender into a 5-by-7-inch drawstring bag and pull the drawstring to seal.

STRESS

Relaxing Catnip Tea Blend

The ingredients in this blend work together to relax and soothe. They make a pretty blend, too. I like to make sure the experience of the tea complements the desired effect. Use a beautiful cup; sit in a favorite chair—whatever makes you feel pampered and calm. This enhances the herbal properties, and besides, you deserve it.

MAKES 12 (1-CUP) SERVINGS

¼ cup dried catnip
3 tablespoons dried
  lemon balm
3 tablespoons dried
  chamomile flowers
1 tablespoon dried
  rose petals

1. In an 8-ounce jar, combine the catnip, lemon balm, chamomile, and rose. Label and date the jar.

2. To use, put 2 rounded teaspoons of loose tea in an infuser and place it in a 10-ounce mug. Cover with boiling water and steep for 5 to 10 minutes. Remove the infuser. Compost the solids.

3. Store the loose tea in a cool place out of direct sunlight for up to 1 year.

Relaxing Passionflower Infusion

When you're feeling stressed, you'll find this relaxing passionflower infusion brings an almost instant sense of calm. Some people become quite sleepy after enjoying this infusion, so be sure you know how it will affect you before driving, operating machinery, or doing tasks that require your full attention.

MAKES 10 DOSES

2 cups dried
   passionflower
1 cup dried
   chamomile flowers
1 cup dried lemon balm
½ cup dried catnip
¼ cup dried
   lavender flowers
2 cups water (per dose)
Raw honey or stevia, for
   sweetening (optional)

1. In a large bowl, combine the passionflower, chamomile flowers, lemon balm, catnip, and lavender. Transfer to an airtight container. Label and date it.

2. To use, in a medium saucepan, combine ½ cup of the herbal mixture with the water and bring the mixture to a boil over medium-high heat.

3. Reduce the heat to medium-low and allow the infusion to simmer for about 15 minutes. Remove the pan from the heat.

4. Strain into a mug, using the back of a spoon to press the liquid from the herbs before composting them. Sweeten the tea with honey (if using).

5. Store the loose tea in a cool place out of direct sunlight for up to 1 year.

Seaweed, Salt, and Lavender Bath

Thalassotherapy is another name for seaweed bath therapy. Some say that humans came from the sea, and the minerals found in seaweed and sea salt in warm water are terrific for skin issues like eczema and psoriasis. This bath is

CONTINUED »

a great way to enjoy the soothing benefits of oceanic plants without the sharks or jellyfish!

MAKES 10 BATHS

2 cups dried seaweed
(bladder wrack,
nori, and kelp are all
good choices)
1 cup dried
lavender flowers
2 cups sea salt
1 to 2 quarts water

1. In a large bowl, combine the seaweed, lavender, and salt. Transfer to a half-gallon glass container or a quart jar and a smaller jar.

2. Measure ½ cup and pour it into a muslin bag.

3. Heat the water to just boiling, then remove from the heat.

4. Soak the bag in the hot water while running a very warm bath.

5. Pour the hot tea and the bag into the tub.

6. Store the remaining bath salts in a labeled, dated, airtight container between uses. The bath salts will last for up to 1 year.

TENSION

Emotional Support Tonic

These herbs help support and condition your overworked nervous system and adrenal glands. The nettle is extracted in vinegar to obtain more of the minerals, while the others are alcohol-based tinctures. The honey adds sweetness. Depending on how you want to use this tonic (it makes a delicious salad dressing), you may choose not to add the honey.

MAKES 4 CUPS

2½ cups
nettle-infused vinegar

4 tablespoons
eleuthero tincture
2 tablespoons
ashwagandha tincture

2 tablespoons
astragalus tincture
½ cup raw
honey (optional)

CONTINUED »

1. In a 1-quart glass jar, combine the vinegar, eleuthero, ashwagandha, and astralagus tinctures, and honey (if using). Cover and shake well to dissolve the honey. Label the jar accordingly.

2. Using a dropper, take 1½ dropperfuls (38 drops) in the earlier part of the day, either added to a small glass of water or straight.

3. Store the tonic at room temperature. It will last indefinitely.

TENSION

Head and Shoulders Tension Tincture

When you are stressed, you clench your jaw, hunch your shoulders toward your ears, and keep your tongue tight to the top of your mouth. After a while, this can result in a sore jaw, possibly chipped teeth, and a painful neck and shoulders. This tincture can ease tension and promote relaxation.

MAKES 2 OUNCES

2 tablespoons
skullcap tincture

1 tablespoon
passionflower tincture

1½ teaspoons
valerian tincture

1½ teaspoons blue
vervain tincture

2 tablespoons water or
juice (per dose)

1. In a 1-cup glass measuring cup, combine the skullcap, passionflower, valerian, and blue vervain tinctures.

2. Transfer the mixture to a 2-ounce dropper bottle.

3. Label and date the tincture blend.

4. Take 1 dropperful (25 drops) in the water or juice as needed. Repeat the dose 30 minutes later if needed.

5. Store the tincture blend in a cool, dark place for up to 3 years.

Nighttime Snack-O

This combination is good for all ages. Gelatin desserts are 97 to 99 percent protein, and they may relieve joint pain and improve brain function. Not a bad snack!

MAKES 4 SERVINGS

2 cups water

1 tablespoon dried
passionflower

1 tablespoon dried
chamomile flowers

1 tablespoon dried
lemon balm

1 6-ounce package
gelatin dessert mix,
any flavor, regular
or sugar-free

1. In a saucepan, bring the water to a boil over high heat.

2. Put the passionflower, chamomile, and lemon balm in a muslin bag, close the bag, and lower it into the boiling water.

3. Remove the pan from the heat and let steep for 20 minutes, then remove the bag, giving it a good squeeze. Compost the solids.

4. There should be close to 2 cups of tea. No need to add water to make up the difference. Use this liquid to make the gelatin dessert, using the instructions on the package.

5. Serve about an hour before bedtime. It also makes a good "cooldown" dessert in situations where people are overstimulated.

6. Refrigerate unused portions for up to a week.

Peace Melt and Pour Soap

Aromatherapy can make huge shifts in our mood or emotions. Soap is a great way to make use of that therapy. It can be something as small as washing the hands or as grand as washing the entire body. Some people

CONTINUED »

don't like the scent of patchouli. In blends, patchouli takes the backseat and works as a fixative for the other oils. However, some may prefer clary sage as a substitute.

MAKES 4 BARS (4 OUNCES EACH)

1 pound melt and pour (glycerin) soap
1 teaspoon patchouli essential oil
1 teaspoon neroli essential oil

1. Chop the soap base into small chunks and place them in a large microwave-safe measuring cup. Heat in the microwave in 30-second bursts, stirring in between, until the soap is almost completely melted. Alternatively, you can melt it into a double boiler on the stovetop.

2. When the soap still has a few pea-size solid parts floating, remove it from the heat and stir in the patchouli and neroli essential oils.

3. Pour the liquid into molds. Muffin tins lined with paper liners work well for this.

4. Wrap any bars you don't plan to use immediately in plastic, and label them. They will keep indefinitely in a cool, dry place.

TENSION

Unwind Syrup

I find this blend to be so comforting and versatile that it's become a go-to in our house. Not only are the herbs relaxing and calming, but they also improve digestion. This is just the thing you need when it's hard to leave behind work or school worries. Keeping it available as syrup means that a teaspoon or three can be added to teas or served over ice cream, oatmeal, or pieces of cut fresh fruit.

CONTINUED »

MAKES 8 OUNCES

½ **cup dried mint**
½ **cup dried**
  chamomile flowers
2 **tablespoons dried**
  lavender flowers
½ **cup raw honey**

1. In a small saucepan, combine the mint, chamomile, and lavender. Set aside.

2. In a separate pan over high heat, boil enough water to just cover the herb mixture. Pour the boiling water over the herbs, cover, and steep for 4 to 8 hours or overnight.

3. Strain into a small saucepan and compost the solids.

4. Heat the strained tea over medium-low heat until it reaches a simmer.

5. Measure ½ cup of the liquid. If there is less than ½ cup, add very hot water to make up the difference. If there is more than ½ cup, either simmer to reduce or discard the excess.

6. Add the honey and mix well to combine. Pour into a glass jar, and label and date it accordingly.

7. This syrup can keep up to 4 months in a cool, dry place, or up to 1 year in the refrigerator.

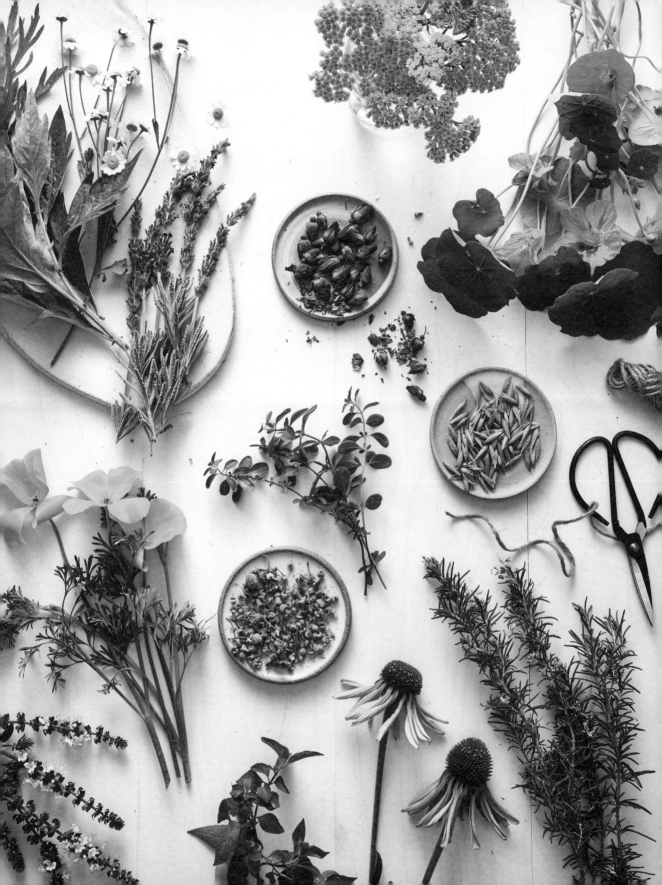

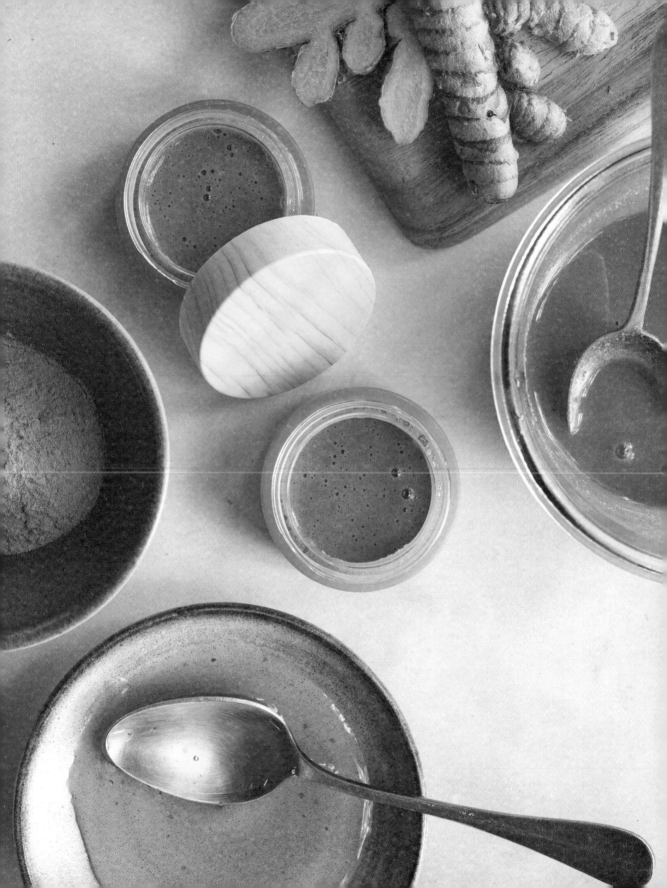

CHAPTER SEVEN

Remedies for Skin and Beauty

Our skin is an incredibly versatile organ. We don't even notice how hard it works for us. Food or medicine allergens show up as hives or welts as the skin works to remove them from our systems. Brush against poison ivy or get too much sun, and the skin reacts quickly to keep out the toxins and prevent infection.

As our largest organ, our skin deserves some attention and assistance. You can create simple, pure remedies for many of the blemishes, rashes, and dryness that tax your valiant defender. In this chapter, you'll find a carefully selected array of useful, delightful, skin-loving potions and concoctions that will keep that skin glowing.

Juniper Berry–Lavender Toner

This facial toner is simple but powerful. The essential oils offer a pleasant aroma, plus they are mighty antiseptics that stimulate your circulation and help damaged skin heal.

MAKES 30 TREATMENTS

½ cup alcohol-free witch hazel hydrosol

4 drops juniper berry essential oil

4 drops lavender essential oil

1. In a dark-colored glass bottle, combine the witch hazel, juniper berry essential oil, and lavender essential oil.

2. Cap tightly and shake well. Label and date the bottle.

3. Using a cotton ball, apply a thin layer to your freshly washed face. Follow up with oil-free moisturizer.

4. Use this toner morning and evening.

5. Store in a cool, dark place for up to 1 month.

Lavender Bath Salt

Epsom salts are a well-known folk remedy for body acne for good reason. They ease inflammation and help purge toxins. Lavender's natural antiseptic properties stop bacteria in their tracks.

MAKES 1 CUP

1 cup Epsom salts

20 drops lavender essential oil

1. In a medium bowl, combine the Epsom salts and 5 drops of lavender essential oil. Blend using a whisk or fork.

2. Add 5 more drops of lavender essential oil and mix well.

CONTINUED »

3. Repeat the process until all 20 drops of the essential oil have been mixed in.

4. Using a funnel, transfer the bath salt to a glass jar with a tight-fitting lid. Label and date the jar.

5. To use, mix ¼ cup of the bath salt into a comfortably warm bath.

6. Soak for at least 15 minutes. Use as often as you like.

7. Store in a cool, dry place for up to 3 months.

ACNE

Lavender Scar Salve

Lavender, rose hip seed oil, cocoa butter, and beeswax come together in this soothing, healing scar salve. Apply it to new scars to prevent them from becoming tough and put it on older scars to help soften their appearance.

MAKES 60 DOSES

¼ **cup cocoa butter**
1 **teaspoon finely grated beeswax**
1 **tablespoon rose hip seed oil**
20 **drops lavender essential oil**

1. In a medium saucepan, combine the cocoa butter and beeswax. Warm over low to medium-low heat just until the beeswax melts.

2. Stir well and remove the pan from the heat. Add the rose hip seed oil and lavender essential oil, stirring again to ensure that all the ingredients are mixed well.

3. Pour the salve into a wide-mouthed container and allow it to cool completely before capping, labeling, and dating.

4. Coat the affected areas completely 1 to 3 times a day.

5. Store in a cool, dark place for up to 1 year.

ACNE

Peppermint–Tea Tree Toner

Soften your skin while eliminating acne with this antibacterial toner. The olive oil it contains helps keep skin supple, while the tea tree oil and peppermint oil penetrate pimples.

MAKES 30 DOSES

¼ **cup olive oil**

15 **drops tea tree essential oil**

5 **drops peppermint essential oil**

1. In a dark-colored glass bottle with a narrow neck, combine the olive oil with the tea tree and peppermint essential oils. Cap tightly and shake well. Label and date the jar.

2. Using a cotton ball, apply the toner to your entire face up to 3 times a day. Leave it in place for 10 minutes, then rinse with cool water.

3. Store in a cool, dark place for up to 1 year.

ACNE

Rosemary–Mint Facial Scrub

By exfoliating gently, this facial scrub helps unblock clogged pores. The white wine and honey soften skin and the rosemary stimulates cell renewal. Use this scrub to stop acne outbreaks fast.

MAKES 1 TREATMENT

½ **teaspoon chopped fresh mint leaves**

½ **teaspoon fresh rosemary leaves**

½ **teaspoon fresh thyme leaves**

2 **tablespoons white wine**

1 **teaspoon raw honey**

2 **teaspoons fine sea salt**

1. In a small saucepan, combine the mint, rosemary, thyme, white wine, and honey.

2. Turn the heat to medium-high and bring to a simmer.

CONTINUED »

3. Reduce the heat to medium-low and simmer for 10 minutes or until the volume has been reduced by half.

4. Allow the mixture to cool completely.

5. Transfer the liquid to a small glass bowl.

6. Add the sea salt and stir gently.

7. Using gentle circular motions, apply the scrub to your freshly washed face. Leave in place for 5 to 10 minutes.

8. Rinse your face with cool water and pat dry. Follow up with oil-free moisturizer.

9. Use this scrub twice weekly during acne breakouts.

ACNE

Soothing Aloe Vera and Calendula Facial

Calendula is a gentle astringent that eliminates bacteria while easing inflammation. This soothing facial stops redness and relieves discomfort while restoring skin's balance and improving your complexion.

MAKES 1 TREATMENT

½ teaspoon alcohol-free
  aloe vera gel
½ teaspoon calendula-
  infused oil (page 30)
1 drop chamomile
  essential oil

1. In a small bowl, combine the aloe vera gel, calendula-infused oil, and chamomile essential oil.

2. Using your fingertips, apply a thin layer to your freshly washed face.

3. Leave in place for 5 to 10 minutes.

CONTINUED »

4. Rinse your face with cool water and pat dry.

5. Repeat this treatment once daily while acne persists. Follow up with your favorite oil-free moisturizer, if needed.

ACNE

Tea Tree Body Wash

Tea tree essential oil is a powerful antibacterial, yet safe for use on blemished skin and effective at easing inflammation and redness. Raw honey smooths skin texture and fast-tracks the healing process.

MAKES ABOUT 1 CUP

⅔ cup unscented liquid castile soap
¼ cup raw honey
2 teaspoons sesame oil
60 drops tea tree essential oil

1. In a medium bowl, whisk together the liquid castile soap, honey, and sesame oil.

2. Add the tea tree essential oil and whisk again, stirring for 30 seconds to ensure that all the ingredients are well incorporated.

3. Using a funnel, transfer the body wash to a plastic squeeze bottle. An empty, clean shampoo bottle also works well. Label and date it.

4. In the shower or tub, squirt a dime-size amount of body wash onto a bath pouf, washcloth, or bathing brush.

5. Gently scrub your body, paying close attention to the areas where acne is prevalent. Leave in place for 5 to 10 minutes before rinsing with water.

6. Store in a cool, dark place for up to 3 months.

Lavender–Witch Hazel Freshening Wipes

With these wipes, you can freshen up between showers, post-gym, or before a stressful meeting. They kill bacteria in an instant. You can buy a bag of cotton cosmetic pads at your local drug store or supermarket for just a few dollars, and you'll use them to make the wipes in this recipe. Both the lavender and witch hazel stop stink fast.

MAKES 20 WIPES

½ **cup alcohol-free witch hazel hydrosol**
20 drops lavender essential oil

1. In a glass jar, combine the witch hazel and lavender essential oil.

2. Swirl the jar for about 30 seconds to combine the ingredients.

3. Stack 20 cotton cosmetic pads in the jar.

4. Cap tightly with a lid and shake the jar gently to ensure that all the pads are soaked with the solution. Label and date the jar.

5. Swab underarms and other smelly areas as needed. Store in a cool place out of direct sunlight, where it will last for up to 1 month.

Natural Rosemary-Mint Deodorant

Aluminum and other chemicals in commercially produced deodorants can be harmful to your health. Eliminate body odor naturally and enjoy healthy, moisturized skin with this delightfully scented rosemary-mint deodorant.

CONTINUED »

MAKES 60 DOSES

¾ cup baking soda

¾ cup arrowroot powder

1 cup coconut oil

15 drops rosemary
  essential oil

15 drops mint
  essential oil

1. In a medium glass bowl, combine the baking soda and arrowroot powder. Add the coconut oil, using a pastry blender or fork to thoroughly mix it with the dry ingredients.

2. Add the rosemary and mint essential oils, blending thoroughly.

3. Transfer the deodorant to a wide-mouth jar with a tight-fitting lid. Label and date the jar.

4. Store in the refrigerator when the indoor temperature reaches 76°F or higher, since the coconut oil will melt when warmed. This deodorant will keep for up to 1 year.

BODY ODOR

Shower Steamers

These are very much like bath bombs, but they are used in the shower and contain penetrating essential oils.

MAKES 4 TREATMENTS

30 drops peppermint
  essential oil

30 drops eucalyptus
  essential oil

30 drops rosemary
  essential oil

1 cup baking soda

½ cup citric acid

2 tablespoons cornstarch
  or arrowroot powder

About ¼ cup alcohol-free
  witch hazel hydrosol in
  a spray bottle

1. In a small bowl, mix together the peppermint, eucalyptus, and rosemary essential oils.

2. In a medium bowl, mix together the baking soda, citric acid, and cornstarch. Spray the powder mixture with the witch hazel with one hand, and continue mixing with the other hand until the

CONTINUED »

mixture holds together like damp sand. Add the essential oil mixture and work it in with your hand.

3. Fill molds of your choice. You can allow them to dry for a day in the molds (and another day out of the mold), or you can remove them after a couple of minutes and allow them to air dry for a day or two.

4. Place a dried tablet at the edge of where water hits in the shower so it just barely gets wet. It will release its scent slowly as you shower.

5. Store extra shower steamers in an airtight container, and label and date the container accordingly. Store in a cool, dry place, and use within 1 year.

BRITTLE NAILS

Aloe Vera and Geranium Nail Soak

With protein-rich gelatin to strengthen nails naturally, this soothing soak also contains aloe vera and geranium for soft, smooth skin.

MAKES 1 TREATMENT

1 tablespoon
  unflavored gelatin
½ cup boiling water
1 tablespoon
  alcohol-free aloe
  vera gel
4 drops geranium
  essential oil

1. In a large wide bowl, combine the gelatin and water. With a spoon or whisk, stir until the gelatin dissolves completely. Let cool until the mixture is comfortably warm.

2. Stir in the aloe vera gel and geranium essential oil.

3. Immerse your hands in the mixture and let them soak for 5 to 10 minutes.

CONTINUED »

4. When the water cools, remove your hands and pat them dry with a towel. Follow up with your favorite moisturizer.

5. Repeat once weekly for strong nails that resist cracking and peeling.

BUG PROBLEMS

Catnip and Rose Geranium Bug Repelling Spray

The botanicals in this natural bug spray are as effective as harsh chemicals, without the dangerous side effects. In recent years, ticks and mosquitoes have been found to carry new diseases, so avoiding their bites is more important than ever.

MAKES ABOUT 1 QUART

For the alcohol

2 cups finely chopped blooming fresh catnip

1 cup finely chopped fresh rose geranium leaves

1 cup chopped lemongrass

½ cup dried lavender flowers

1 quart 80- or 100-proof vodka

For the oil

1 cup olive oil

2 tablespoons chopped blooming fresh catnip

2 tablespoons chopped fresh rose geranium leaves

2 tablespoons chopped lemongrass

2 tablespoons dried lavender flowers

30 drops lemon eucalyptus essential oil

To make the alcohol

1. Place the catnip, rose geranium, lemongrass, and lavender in a jar and cover with the vodka. Let steep at room temperature for 2 weeks.

2. Strain and return the liquid to the jar. Compost the solids.

CONTINUED »

3. In a baking dish, combine the olive oil, catnip, rose geranium, lemongrass, and lavender. Put in the oven at the lowest setting (180°F to 200°F, generally labeled "warm") for 2 hours.

4. Strain the oil into a large measuring cup and cool to room temperature.

To make the spray

5. Fill spray bottles with one part oil and two parts alcohol, using a funnel if necessary.

6. To use, spray directly onto skin. Shake vigorously between uses to be sure the alcohol and oil combine for a longer-lasting repellent. Store in a cool, dry place out of direct sunlight, where it will last indefinitely.

CELLULITE

Smoothing Rosemary-Geranium Cellulite Scrub

Rosemary and geranium essential oils help tone and smooth skin while increasing circulation. This scrub should be used each day in the shower for best results; at the same time, focus on exercising problem areas to tighten underlying muscle layers and eliminate cellulite from the inside out.

CONTINUED »

MAKES 4 TO 8 DOSES

½ **cup cocoa butter**
½ **cup sugar**
20 **drops rosemary**
    essential oil
20 **drops geranium**
    essential oil

1. In a small bowl, combine the cocoa butter and sugar. Add the rosemary and geranium essential oils and stir again, ensuring that all the ingredients are mixed well.

2. Transfer the mixture to a glass jar with a tight-fitting lid. Label, date, and store it in a cool, dark place for up to 1 year.

CHAPPED LIPS

Lavender-Frankincense Lip Balm

Natural emollients and healing essential oils come together in this soothing lip balm. It is also an excellent balm for applying to dry, cracked skin on hands and feet.

MAKES 30 DOSES

1 **tablespoon olive oil**
1½ **teaspoons**
    avocado oil
1½ **teaspoons jojoba oil**
1½ **teaspoons finely**
    grated beeswax
5 **drops lavender**
    essential oil
5 **drops frankincense**
    (boswellia)
    essential oil

1. In a medium saucepan, combine the olive oil, avocado oil, jojoba oil, and beeswax over low to medium-low heat, warming just until the beeswax melts. Mix thoroughly and remove the saucepan from the heat. Allow the mixture to cool for a minute while stirring, and add the lavender and frankincense essential oils.

2. Transfer the lip balm to a small glass container and cool completely. Cover, label, and date the balm.

3. Using your index finger, apply a thin layer to your lips.

4. Store in a cool, dark place for up to 6 months.

Lavender-Geranium Lip Balm

You'll love how silky soft your lips feel as this healing balm boosts hydration and soothes irritation. The lavender and geranium essential oils help damaged skin heal while leaving a hint of pleasant fragrance.

MAKES 30 TREATMENTS

1 tablespoon beeswax

1 tablespoon coconut oil

1 teaspoon calendula-infused oil (page 30)

2 drops lavender essential oil

1 drop geranium essential oil

1. In a double boiler, combine the beeswax and coconut oil over low heat. Stir gently until the beeswax has melted completely.

2. Remove the pan from the heat and add the calendula-infused oil. Stir well. Add the lavender and geranium essential oils and stir well.

3. Pour the balm into a small jar and let cool completely. Cover, label, and date the balm.

4. Using your index finger, apply a thin layer to your lips.

5. Store in a cool, dark place for up to 6 months.

Lemon Balm Lip Saver

Once the lips become chapped, you need an emollient balm for true healing. The allantoin in comfrey is amazing, and lemon balm has many healing properties that also help fight fever blisters.

CONTINUED »

MAKES ABOUT 4 OUNCES

3 tablespoons
  coconut oil
1 tablespoon dried
  comfrey leaf
  (preferably
  not powdered)
1 tablespoon dried
  lemon balm
  (preferably
  not powdered)
1 tablespoon
  cocoa butter
1½ tablespoons beeswax

1. In a small saucepan over medium-low heat, warm the coconut oil until it melts, then stir in the comfrey and lemon balm. Keep heating the oil to just below a simmer. You may heat it and then remove it from the heat for 10 minutes, and repeat this several times until it has been heated for a good hour.

2. Remove the pan from the heat and allow the mixture to steep for another hour.

3. Strain into a small bowl. (Expect to lose a tablespoon of oil to the herbs.)

4. Return the strained oil to the saucepan. Add the cocoa butter and beeswax to the warm coconut oil and heat over low heat to melt it all together.

5. Stir well, then pour the liquid balm into labeled containers. Store in a cool, dry place and use within 6 to 9 months.

6. This is quite shelf stable, but it can melt in hot weather. If it does, put the closed container in the refrigerator and it'll be as good as new.

DANDRUFF

Ginger–Tea Tree Scalp Tonic

Ginger's anti-inflammatory action eases the itching associated with dandruff. Olive oil imparts natural moisture to dry, flaky skin. Tea tree essential oil lends a hand by killing fungus.

MAKES 1 TREATMENT

1 (palm-size) piece fresh
  ginger, peeled

1 tablespoon olive oil
2 drops tea tree
  essential oil

CONTINUED »

1. Use a garlic press or juicer to extract as much juice from the ginger as you can.

2. In a small bowl, combine the ginger juice, olive oil, and tea tree essential oil.

3. Wet your hair and apply the entire remedy to the scalp. Massage gently, then leave the treatment in place for 15 minutes.

4. When finished, rinse your hair thoroughly with cool water. Follow up with your favorite shampoo and conditioner.

5. Repeat this treatment 2 or 3 times weekly until the dandruff is gone. If you use a hair dryer, avoid exposing your scalp to high heat, as that slows the healing process.

DANDRUFF

Herbal Dandruff Shampoo

This natural dandruff shampoo is a fantastic alternative to commercial preparations, thanks to a cocktail of high-powered, antioxidant-rich herbs that heal the scalp without the signature medicinal scent of over-the-counter options.

MAKES 15 TREATMENTS

1 cup water
1 heaping tablespoon
  dried lavender flowers
1 heaping tablespoon
  dried mint

1 heaping tablespoon
  dried rosemary
⅓ cup liquid castile soap
¼ teaspoon almond oil
  or olive oil

5 drops eucalyptus
  essential oil
5 drops tea tree
  essential oil

CONTINUED »

1. In a small saucepan, bring the water to a boil over high heat. Add the lavender, mint, and rosemary, cover the pan, and reduce the heat to low. Simmer for 20 minutes.

2. Strain the liquid into a bowl and compost the solids. Let the mixture cool.

3. Add the castile soap and mix gently. Add the almond oil and eucalyptus and tea tree essential oils. Mix gently, then use a funnel to transfer the shampoo to a bottle. Label and date the bottle.

4. Shampoo and follow up with your favorite conditioner. Style as usual, avoiding high heat from the blow-dryer.

5. Use daily whenever dandruff is a problem. Store in the shower. Use within 2 months.

DANDRUFF

Rosemary Scalp Tonic

Rosemary has a pleasant, uplifting fragrance, and its antibacterial and antifungal properties make it an excellent treatment for dandruff. Borax is also renowned for its ability to help clear dandruff naturally; look for a brand that contains no additives. If using fresh rosemary, store the tonic in the refrigerator; it will keep for up to one week. If using dried rosemary, store in a cool, dark place or refrigerate if preferred; it will keep for up to one month.

MAKES 50 DOSES

4 cups water

1 cup chopped fresh rosemary leaves,

or 2 cups crumbled dried rosemary

½ cup borax

CONTINUED »

1. In a medium saucepan, combine the water and rosemary and bring the mixture to a boil over medium-high heat.

2. Reduce the heat to medium-low and allow the mixture to simmer for 15 to 20 minutes, until the liquid reduces by half. Strain into a jar or bowl, using the back of a spoon to press as much liquid from the rosemary as possible. Compost the solids.

3. Add the borax, stirring to dissolve. When the tonic is completely cool, transfer it to a clean spray bottle. Label and date it.

4. With either wet or dry hair, spritz your scalp thoroughly. Massage gently, then leave the treatment in place for 30 seconds.

5. When finished, rinse your hair thoroughly with cool water. Follow up with your favorite shampoo and conditioner.

6. Repeat this treatment 2 to 3 times weekly until the dandruff is gone. If you use a hair dryer, avoid exposing your scalp to high heat, as that slows the healing process.

DERMATITIS

Cooling Aloe Vera Gel with Witch Hazel

This quick gel eases the discomfort of hot, itchy dermatitis in less time than it takes to make. For maximum results, take a hot bath or shower

CONTINUED »

*right before application to open pores and allow the treatment to
penetrate faster.*

MAKES 1 TREATMENT

1 tablespoon
  alcohol-free aloe
  vera gel
½ teaspoon alcohol-free
  witch hazel hydrosol

1. In a small bowl, combine the aloe vera gel and witch hazel. Blend with a whisk or fork.

2. Using your fingers or a cotton pad, apply the gel to the affected body part and let it penetrate.

3. Wait a few minutes, then apply a second coat if itching or heat is still present.

4. Reapply every 1 to 2 hours as needed.

5. Store the gel in an airtight container in the refrigerator for up to 3 days.

DIRTY HAIR

Dry Shampoo

*You just have to leave the house for a couple hours to run errands, but the
effort of a shower, getting dressed, driving . . . it's all too much. Dry shampoo
can freshen the appearance of hair enough to pull off not showering for a little
while longer. The measurements in this recipe are flexible. If your hair is dark,
use more powdered herbs and less arrowroot powder.*

**MAKES 5 TO 10 APPLICATIONS
(DEPENDING ON HAIR LENGTH)**

¼ cup arrowroot
  powder (or any kind of
  body powder)
1 heaping tablespoon
  powdered mint
1 heaping tablespoon
  powdered lavender

1. In a measuring cup, combine the arrowroot, mint, and lavender. Mix the ingredients very well and transfer into a small, labeled jar, ideally with a shaker top. Store in a cool, dark place out of direct sunlight for up to 1 year.

2. Place a scant teaspoon of the mixture in the palm of one hand and distribute over both palms.

CONTINUED »

3. Lightly massage it into the hair, particularly near the scalp. It will absorb excess oil and give the hair volume.

4. Brush thoroughly.

5. Wash your hair before going to bed, because the dry shampoo will weigh the hair down and may leave it feeling gunky the next day.

Morning Mint Dry Shampoo

In between shampoos, dry shampoo can give your hair an extra day by sopping up oil. When I was in school, some of my classmates used baby powder. This is better.

MAKES 1 CUP

3 ounces cornstarch
3 ounces arrowroot powder
1 ounce baking soda
½ ounce powdered mint
½ ounce orris root powder
30 drops peppermint essential oil
30 drops spearmint essential oil

1. In a small bowl, whisk together the cornstarch, arrowroot, baking soda, mint, orris root, peppermint oil, and spearmint oil, making sure the essential oils don't clump together and are well distributed in the powders.

2. Sprinkle 1 or 2 teaspoons of the powder on your scalp and gently tussle it into your hair.

3. Let sit for 5 or 10 minutes. Brush through and style.

4. If you can, find a powder shaker for storage. Repurposed Parmesan cheese jars work well, too. Label and date the container. Store in a cool, dry place, and use within 2 years.

DRY HAIR

Lavender Hair Mask

Yogurt, honey, and rich oils infuse protein and moisture into parched hair, repairing damage while amping up shine. Prepare this treatment just before you shampoo.

MAKES 1 TREATMENT

¼ cup plain yogurt

1 tablespoon raw honey

1 tablespoon olive oil or sunflower oil

5 drops lavender essential oil

1. In a blender, combine yogurt, honey, olive or sunflower oil, and lavender oil. Process on medium-low speed until blended.

2. Transfer the mixture to a plastic squeeze bottle.

3. Work the treatment through your freshly shampooed hair, and massage it into your scalp. Leave the mask in place for 15 minutes, then rinse with water.

4. Use twice weekly for best results.

DRY HAIR

Rosemary Hair Repair

The protein in gelatin fortifies damaged hair, while apple cider vinegar and rosemary give it lustrous shine. Prepare this treatment just before you shampoo.

MAKES 1 TREATMENT

1 cup hot tap water

1 tablespoon unflavored gelatin

1 teaspoon apple cider vinegar

5 drops rosemary essential oil

1. In a small bowl, combine the water and gelatin, whisking to blend well. Set the mixture aside for about 5 minutes.

CONTINUED »

2. Once the mixture begins to gel slightly, add the vinegar and rosemary essential oil. Stir well to combine.

3. Work the treatment through your freshly shampooed hair and into your scalp, then leave it in place for 10 minutes.

4. Rinse with warm water.

5. Repeat once or twice weekly for best results.

DRY HANDS

Pampering Chamomile-Lavender Scrub

If your hands are feeling dry and looking overworked, treat them to a quick pick-me-up. This thick, rich sugar scrub exfoliates and moisturizes, leaving skin feeling refreshed. Try it on dry feet, knees, and elbows, too.

MAKES 6 OUNCES

6 tablespoons sugar
1 ounce beeswax, grated
¼ cup olive oil
4 drops chamomile essential oil
2 drops lavender essential oil

1. Put the sugar in a small jar.

2. In a double boiler over low heat, combine the beeswax and olive oil. Stir gently until the beeswax has completely melted. Remove the pan from the heat and let the mixture cool for 2 minutes.

3. Pour the olive oil and beeswax blend into the jar on top of the sugar, and allow the mixture to cool for 5 minutes.

4. Stir in the chamomile and lavender essential oils and cap the jar tightly. Label and date the jar.

CONTINUED »

5. Gently massage your hands with 1 teaspoon of the scrub for at least 1 minute, then rinse with warm water. Follow up with your favorite moisturizer.

6. Use 3 times weekly for soft, smooth hands.

7. Store in a cool, dark place. Use within 6 months.

DRY SCALP

Aloe Hair Mask

Aloe has a reputation for working wonders on damaged hair, soothing itchy scalps, and relieving dandruff. It leaves hair smooth and shiny. The oil and milk in this mask increase these actions, and the nettle helps strengthen hair and keep it healthy.

MAKES 1 MASK FOR LONG HAIR OR 2 MASKS FOR SHORT HAIR

¼ cup alcohol-free aloe
 vera gel
¼ cup coconut milk
2 tablespoons
 powdered nettles
1 tablespoon coconut oil

1. In a microwave-safe bowl, combine the aloe vera, coconut milk, nettles, and coconut oil and mix until smooth.

2. Warm the mixture in the microwave in 30-second bursts (or in a double boiler for about 3 minutes) until the coconut oil is melted.

3. The mask can be used about once a week. Work it through dry hair and into the scalp and spend a few minutes massaging it in. Cover hair with a shower cap or plastic wrap, then cover with a towel to retain the heat. Let the mask sit for about 30 minutes, then rinse, condition, and admire.

4. Store in a labeled, dated, airtight jar and refrigerate. Use within 2 weeks.

Rosemary-Mint Scalp and Hair Toner

Wake up in the shower when you massage a spray or two of this bracing toner into your hair and scalp! The massaging action will increase blood flow, and the aromatherapy benefits of both herbs are reviving.

MAKES 10 TO 12 OUNCES

½ **cup water**

1 **tablespoon dried rosemary**

1 **tablespoon dried peppermint**

1 **cup alcohol-free witch hazel hydrosol**

For super-charged toner, add 5 drops each of rosemary and peppermint essential oils to the mix (optional)

1. In a small saucepan, bring the water to a boil over high heat.

2. Remove the pan from the heat. Infuse the water with the rosemary and peppermint and steep for 30 minutes.

3. Strain into a small bowl or glass measuring cup and compost the solids. Allow the liquid to cool. Add the witch hazel and essential oils (if using), and transfer to a spray bottle. Label and date the bottle.

4. After washing the hair, use a few sprays or about a tablespoon of the liquid to wake up the scalp and hair. It isn't necessary to rinse out. It is nice on the face after washing, too.

5. Use within 2 to 3 weeks.

Apres Bath Moisturizing Spray

Very dry skin makes an easy target for bacteria and irritation. It just feels better to have skin that feels like it fits.

CONTINUED »

My sister first made this for my mother when she couldn't reach her back to put lotion on it. Mom didn't want to add oil to the bathtub because it would get too slippery. She liked the spray so much that we've all used it ever since.

MAKES 8 OUNCES

¾ cup water

1 tablespoon pure vegetable glycerin

1 tablespoon jojoba oil

2 tablespoons comfrey tincture

20 drops any essential oil (optional)

1. In a 2-cup glass measuring cup, combine the water, glycerin, jojoba oil, comfrey tincture, and essential oil (if using). Carefully pour the mixture into an 8-ounce spray bottle and cap tightly. Label and date the bottle.

2. Shake well before each use. Spray after showering or bathing, while the skin is still damp.

3. Refrigerate between uses. Remove the spray from the refrigerator 1 hour before showering so it isn't cold. Return to the refrigerator after use, where it can be stored for up to 2 months.

DRY SKIN

Honey Moisture Mask with Hyssop and Lavender

This trio of skin saviors—hyssop, lavender, and honey—soothes irritation, nourishes parched cells, and calms inflammation. Over-the-counter aloe vera gel is a great substitution if you don't have an aloe vera plant.

MAKES 1 TREATMENT

1 aloe vera leaf, or 1 teaspoon store-bought alcohol-free aloe vera gel

1 teaspoon raw honey, warmed

1 teaspoon fresh hyssop leaves, finely chopped

2 drops lavender essential oil

1. Split the aloe vera leaf open lengthwise and scoop out the aloe vera gel.

CONTINUED »

2. In a small bowl, combine the aloe vera gel with the honey.

3. Using a fork or a small whisk, stir well.

4. Add the hyssop leaves and lavender essential oil.

5. Stir again to blend all the ingredients.

6. Using your fingertips, apply the entire mask to your face and neck.

7. Lie back and relax for at least 10 to 15 minutes.

8. Rinse your face with cool water when finished. Follow up with your favorite moisturizer.

9. Enjoy twice weekly for best results.

DRY SKIN

Lavender-Geranium Body Cream

Healing essential oils come together with nourishing emollients in this soothing body cream.

MAKES 30 DOSES

1 cup coconut oil
1 cup cocoa butter
½ cup jojoba oil
½ cup avocado oil
30 drops lavender essential oil
30 drops geranium essential oil

1. In a large saucepan, combine the coconut oil, cocoa butter, jojoba oil, and avocado oil over low to medium-low heat, warming just until the coconut butter melts.

2. Mix thoroughly and remove from the heat.

3. Add the lavender and geranium essential oils and blend thoroughly.

CONTINUED »

4. Pour the mixture into a wide-mouth container. Allow the body cream to cool completely before capping. Label and date the container.

5. Store in a cool, dark place for up to 6 months. By putting the cream in 3 8-ounce jars and refrigerating what isn't being used, its shelf life will be extended to 1 year.

DRY SKIN

Rich Chamomile Facial Cream

With rich oils and beeswax for a smooth, supple feel, this moisturizer makes the most of chamomile's healing ability.

MAKES 30 TREATMENTS

1 teaspoon dried
  chamomile flowers
½ cup boiling water
3 tablespoons
  almond oil
3 tablespoons
  avocado oil
1 tablespoon jojoba oil
1 ounce beeswax
2 teaspoons glycerin
10 drops chamomile
  essential oil
10 drops geranium
  essential oil

1. In a small bowl, combine the chamomile flowers and boiling water. Cover the bowl and steep for 15 minutes.

2. Meanwhile, in the top of a double boiler, combine the almond, avocado, and jojoba oils.

3. Add the beeswax to the oils and stir over low heat until melted. Strain the chamomile-infused water into a small bowl, being careful to keep flower bits out of the liquid. Measure 2 tablespoons of the infusion. Discard any unused portion.

4. Transfer the oil mixture to a medium glass bowl. One drop at a time, add the chamomile infusion to the oil mixture, stirring with a small whisk until it thickens and cools.

CONTINUED »

5. Add the glycerin and mix thoroughly. Add the chamomile and geranium essential oils and mix again.

6. Transfer the cream to a glass jar with a tight-fitting lid. Label and date the jar.

7. With your fingertips, massage a small amount onto your freshly washed face, neck, and chest.

8. Use nightly before bed.

9. Store in a cool, dark place for up to 6 months. By putting the cream in 3 8-ounce jars and refrigerating what isn't being used, its shelf life will be extended to 1 year.

DRY SKIN

Wild Violet Skin Cream

Cooling, soothing, and anti-inflammatory, this cream is a dream.

MAKES 10 TO 12 OUNCES

1 cup fresh violet flowers
⅜ cup violet leaf
   pre-infused hempseed
   oil or apricot kernel oil
½ ounce castor oil
1½ ounces shea butter
½ ounce beeswax
40 to 50 drops violet
   leaf essential oil

1. Place the violet flowers in a heatproof glass measuring cup and pour hot (not yet boiling) water over them. Cover and let steep.

2. Put the oils, shea butter, and beeswax in a double boiler. Warm on medium-low heat until everything melts together (alternatively, heat in the microwave in 30-second bursts).

3. Strain the flower tea and measure 10 to 12 tablespoons of the liquid. Note that both the oils and the tea are at similar temperatures.

CONTINUED »

4. Using a hand mixer (or blender) on low speed, slowly mix the strained violet flower tea into the oil mixture. As the oils start to thicken, add the violet leaf essential oil and increase the speed to high. Mix on high speed until the mixture is thick and creamy. Spoon the cream into airtight containers and seal. Label and date the containers.

5. Slather this mixture over dry skin as needed.

6. Store in a cool, dark place for up to 3 months.

DULL HAIR

Rosemary and Nettle Hair and Scalp Rinse

The vinegar in this rinse brings added protection around the hair cuticle. The rosemary and nettle are stimulating and strengthening, leaving the hair shiny and the scalp healthy.

MAKES ABOUT 1 QUART (ABOUT 8 USES, DEPENDING ON LENGTH OF HAIR)

1 quart apple cider vinegar

1 cup fresh rosemary leaves, or ⅓ cup dried

1 cup fresh stinging nettles leaves, or ⅓ cup dried

1. Combine the vinegar, rosemary, and stinging nettles in a large jar. Cover and let steep at room temperature for 3 weeks. Alternatively, you can combine everything in a slow cooker and steep for 4 to 6 hours on low.

2. After steeping, strain the liquid into a quart jar, pressing as much of the vinegar out of the herbs as possible. Compost the solids.

3. To use, after washing your hair, work ½ cup of the rinse (for medium-length hair) through your hair and into the scalp. Rinse well. Any vinegar smell will vanish as your hair dries.

4. Store in the jar at room temperature and use within 1 year.

Shine-On Hair Rinse

Depression feels dull. Personally, when I'm down, it seems like the intensity of my senses has been turned way down—a lot like when I have a bad cold. It is always surprising how much better everything feels when I'm cleaned up and presentable. This rinse is a simple bit of self-care that restores shine by smoothing the outer surface of the hair.

MAKES 3 APPLICATIONS

½ **cup dried rosemary**
½ **cup dried
  lavender flowers**
2½ **cups water**
2 **cups apple
  cider vinegar**

1. In a large heatproof bowl or wide-mouth quart jar, combine the rosemary and lavender.

2. Boil the water and pour it over the herb mixture. Let steep for 1 hour.

3. Strain the liquid into a clean quart jar and stir in the vinegar. Compost the solids. Label and date the jar.

4. After washing your hair, apply 2 cups of the hair rinse. Rinse out with fresh water.

5. Store the remaining hair rinse in an airtight container and use within 1 month.

Chamomile-Aloe Body Oil

Aloe vera gel cools itching and stinging while promoting healing, and chamomile essential oil soothes and moisturizes dry patches. Though this remedy is a simple one, it is wonderfully effective and is safe for children.

CONTINUED »

MAKES 15 DOSES

4 tablespoons
  alcohol-free aloe
  vera gel
2 tablespoons wheat
  germ oil
10 drops chamomile
  essential oil

1. In a small bowl, whisk together the aloe vera gel and wheat germ oil. Add the chamomile essential oil and whisk again, ensuring all the ingredients have been thoroughly incorporated.

2. Apply the balm to eczema patches as needed, refrigerating the balm in an airtight, labeled, and dated container between uses for up to 1 week.

ECZEMA

Chamomile Facial Compress

Instant relief! This soothing compress is a quick, easy remedy that eases discomfort quickly. Chamomile essential oil helps stop inflammation and itching while promoting faster healing.

MAKES 1 TREATMENT

½ cup hot tap water
1 teaspoon coconut oil
6 drops chamomile
  essential oil

1. In a medium shallow bowl, combine the hot tap water and coconut oil. Add the chamomile essential oil and stir.

2. Soak a soft cloth in the mixture and squeeze out the excess liquid.

3. Place the cloth over your face and rest for 15 minutes, refreshing the cloth with the warm solution each time it cools.

4. Apply once or twice daily. Use for as many days as eczema persists.

Soothing Patchouli Eczema Plaster

Patchouli grows best in warm climates. Luckily, it's easy to obtain in the form of essential oil. This plaster soothes eczema while imparting an intoxicating fragrance.

MAKES ABOUT 1 CUP

½ cup coconut oil
8 drops patchouli essential oil
¼ cup oat flour
¼ cup olive oil

1. In a small saucepan, melt the coconut oil over medium-low heat until it liquefies. Add the patchouli essential oil and the oat flour. Stir until blended. Add the olive oil and mix again, stirring until all the ingredients have been incorporated.

2. Remove the pan from the heat. Pour the plaster into a jar and let it cool completely. Cover with a tight cap. Label and date the jar.

3. Apply a thin layer to the affected area as needed.

4. Keep in a cool, dark place and use within 1 month.

Floral Facial Toner

Toners often have alcohol in them, which can be drying to the face. Without the alcohol, this is a gently balancing toner.

MAKES 12 OUNCES

1 cup boiling water
2 tablespoons dried elderflower
¼ cup dried peach leaves, or peach flower–infused vinegar
¼ cup raspberry-infused vinegar
1 teaspoon raw honey
¼ cup aloe vera juice

CONTINUED »

1. In a small bowl, combine the water and elderflower and let steep for 20 minutes.

2. Strain into a medium bowl. Compost the solids.

3. Add the peach leaves, raspberry-infused vinegar, honey, and aloe vera juice to the strained liquid. Mix well.

4. Pour the toner into a 16-ounce glass bottle and label with the name of the formula and the date made.

5. Apply with a cotton ball to a freshly cleaned face.

6. Store the toner at room temperature for up to 30 days, or refrigerate for longer storage.

FACIAL SKIN ISSUES

Rejuvenating Facial Mask

This facial skin soother allows for substitutions, depending on your skin type and the herbs at your disposal. For dry to normal skin, use any blend of nettle, mint, lemon balm, marshmallow powder, or rose to make up your half cup of dried herbs. For oily skin, use any blend of sage, mint, nettle, or lavender.

MAKES 1 FACIAL MASK

½ **cup dried herbs of your choice**
½ **medium cucumber, peeled and seeded**
2 **tablespoons alcohol-free witch hazel hydrosol**

1. In a blender, combine your custom herb blend, cucumber, and witch hazel. Blend until it forms a fairly uniform paste.

2. Apply a thick layer to your face and relax for 15 minutes. Rinse with warm water and lightly pat dry.

Aloe Vera and Peppermint Hair Mask

Aloe vera provides the moisture that dehydrated or damaged locks so desperately need, while jojoba oil adds shine and peppermint essential oil stimulates circulation in your scalp (read: helps new hair grow).

MAKES 1 TREATMENT

1 tablespoon
  alcohol-free aloe
  vera gel
1 tablespoon jojoba oil
6 drops peppermint
  essential oil

1. In a small bowl, combine the aloe vera gel, jojoba oil, and peppermint essential oil.

2. Apply the entire treatment to your hair and scalp, massaging well. Place a disposable shower cap on your head and leave the treatment in place for 15 minutes.

3. When finished, wash and condition your hair as usual.

4. Use once or twice weekly for best results.

HAIR DAMAGE

Nettle, Rosemary, and Monarda Hot Oil Hair Treatment

Hot oil treatments are a time-honored remedy for dry, lifeless hair and a dry scalp. In the winter when we're inside in heated air, a hot oil treatment returns shine and health to the hair. It can also help with split ends by smoothing the hair shaft. In a randomized, controlled trial published in SKINmed, rosemary oil had the same effect on androgenetic alopecia as minoxidil, except that those using rosemary oil had fewer instances of itching. That was daily dosing, but in any case, rosemary oil is stimulating and healing to the scalp.

CONTINUED »

MAKES ABOUT 6 OUNCES

2 tablespoons
  dried nettles
2 tablespoons
  dried monarda
1 cup olive oil
40 drops rosemary
  essential oil

1. Infuse the nettles and monarda in the olive oil for 2 weeks. Strain into a small jar and compost the solids.

2. Add the rosemary essential oil and stir well. Label and date the jar.

3. Massage ½ to 2 teaspoons into your hair, depending on the hair length, then brush it well to distribute it. Wrap your hair in a towel for about 1 hour, then shampoo as usual.

4. Use 1 or 2 times a month.

5. Store in the refrigerator and use within 1 year.

HAIR LOSS

Nasturtium Tincture (or Hair Rinse)

Nasturtium leaves are the most potent part of the plant before it blooms. This tincture does a good job of preserving the healing properties of those early leaves. Take 1 teaspoon of the tincture up to 3 times a day. To make this recipe as a hair rinse, use vinegar instead of alcohol. The hair rinse is thought to promote hair growth by keeping the scalp healthy and stimulated—pour about ½ cup on your hair immediately after washing, massage in thoroughly, and then rinse.

MAKES 1 PINT

1 cup fresh
  nasturtium leaves
¼ cup fresh
  rosemary leaves
¼ cup fresh stinging
  nettle leaves

2 cups 100-proof vodka
  (or apple cider vinegar
  for the hair rinse)

1. In a pint jar, combine the nasturtium, rosemary, and stinging nettles and cover with the vodka (or vinegar if making a hair rinse).

CONTINUED »

2. Cover and let the mixture steep in a cool, dry place for about 1 month. Check that the herbs are submerged in the liquid a couple of times a day, shaking the jar as necessary to ensure that the herbs are completely saturated.

3. After about a month, run the mixture through a food processor and strain into a jar. Label and date the jar.

4. Both the tincture and the rinse will last indefinitely at room temperature.

HAIR LOSS

Rosemary-Lavender Conditioner

Everyone loses between 20 and 100 strands of hair daily, and people who are stressed or who use chlorinated water often lose more. It is important to keep the scalp well-nourished to prevent excess hair loss and promote healthy hair production, and both rosemary and lavender essential oils are renowned for their ability to do just that. If you are going to use all the conditioner within a month or so, feel free to keep it in the shower. If you are going to store it long-term, put it in a cool, dark place, where it will stay fresh for up to one year.

MAKES 30 DOSES

1 cup cocoa butter
1 cup sunflower oil
30 drops rosemary
  essential oil
15 drops lavender
  essential oil

1. In a medium saucepan, combine the cocoa butter and sunflower oil over low to medium-low heat, warming just until the cocoa butter melts. Stir until the cocoa butter and sunflower oil are completely combined, then add the rosemary and lavender essential oils and stir again.

2. Transfer the mixture to a bottle with a narrow neck. Label and date the bottle.

CONTINUED »

3. Use about 1 tablespoon of conditioner after shampooing. Be sure to massage the conditioner into your scalp and allow it to remain there for 30 seconds before rinsing well with warm water. Dry and style your hair as usual.

HYPERPIGMENTATION

Aloe Vera–Lime Mask

Turns out your grandmother was right: The aloe-and-lime combo does fade dark spots. Together, they lighten excess pigment while sloughing away dead skin and promoting new cell growth.

MAKES 1 TREATMENT

1 tablespoon alcohol-free aloe vera gel

1 teaspoon freshly squeezed lime juice

1. In a small bowl, whisk together the aloe vera gel and lime juice.

2. With your fingertips, apply the entire treatment to your freshly washed face.

3. Cover with a paper spa mask and relax for 25 minutes before rinsing it off.

4. Repeat 3 times weekly.

HYPERPIGMENTATION

Turmeric Facial

You might know turmeric as one of the spices that give Indian dishes their signature flavor. This herb also helps even out skin tone. The downside is that it increases sun sensitivity for a few days after treatment. Be vigilant with

CONTINUED »

sunscreen to prevent burns. Also, because turmeric adheres to the whorls and loops on your fingertips and causes yellowing, it's best to wear disposable latex gloves for this treatment.

MAKES 1 TREATMENT

1 teaspoon
  ground turmeric
1 teaspoon full-fat
  powdered milk
3 teaspoons raw honey

1. In a small bowl, whisk together the turmeric, powdered milk, and honey.

2. With a circular motion, gently scrub your face and other areas affected by hyperpigmentation.

3. After scrubbing, leave the treatment in place for 15 minutes.

4. Rinse your face. Follow up with your favorite cleanser, toner, and moisturizer.

5. Use 3 times weekly until spots have faded.

IRRITATION FROM SHAVING

Citrus, Sage, and Lavender Aftershave

This remedy helps tone skin and close pores after shaving. It has a neutral aroma that's refreshing for everyone.

MAKES 12 TO 16 OUNCES DEPENDING ON HOW MUCH LIQUID IS ABSORBED BY THE HERBS

2 cups alcohol-free
  witch hazel hydrosol

2 tablespoons apple
  cider vinegar
Zest of 1 orange

1 ounce dried sage
1 ounce dried
  lavender flowers

1. In a quart jar, combine the witch hazel, vinegar, orange zest, sage, and lavender and screw on the lid.

CONTINUED »

2. Put the jar somewhere you'll see it often and remember to shake it at least once a day for 2 weeks.

3. Strain into a bottle and compost the solids. Label and date the bottle.

4. Splash this on after shaving your face, neck, or legs! It's also very pleasant to keep in a spray bottle in the refrigerator and spray on your face and neck on hot days.

5. This should stay fresh for several months.

ITCHY, ACHY SKIN

Healing Herbal Tub Tea

All the herbs included in this tea are soothing, healing, and terrific for achy, itchy skin or internal discomfort. Soak in the bath for at least 15 minutes. If a fever is present, keep the water tepid.

MAKES ABOUT 6 CUPS

1 cup dried yarrow
1 cup dried
   lavender flowers
1 cup dried plantain
1 cup dried calendula
1 cup dried rose petals
1 cup dried comfrey

1. In a gallon jar or bag, combine the yarrow, lavender, plantain, calendula, rose, and comfrey and mix well. Label and date the container accordingly, and store it in a cool, dark place for up to 1 year.

2. To use, scoop out about ½ cup of the mixture and put it into a large muslin bag or tie tightly into a washcloth.

3. Put the bag in a large pitcher and fill with very hot water. Let steep for 10 to 15 minutes while you prepare the bath. Pour the infused liquid into the tub, swirl it around, and climb in.

Tea Tree Fungus Fighter

Tea tree essential oil is the most powerful herbal antifungal agent available—in fact, it's so powerful that many commercial products use it as their secret ingredient. While working to eliminate itchy, unsightly nail fungus, keep your nails free of polish.

MAKES 1 DOSE

1 gallon hot water
Tea tree essential
   oil, diluted
   (10 drops essential
   oil to 2 tablespoons
   vinegar or fractionated
   coconut oil)

1. Prepare a footbath by pouring the hot water into a shallow basin. Soak your feet in the water for 10 minutes to soften the nails, then trim them if needed. After drying your feet, apply a generous coating of diluted tea tree essential oil to your nails and cuticles, massaging it in thoroughly.

2. Continue this treatment daily until all thickened yellow nail tissue has grown out and been trimmed off; this may take several months, depending on the severity of the infection.

Rosemary-Lemon Rinse

Rosemary and lemon essential oils and apple cider vinegar cut through excess oil, nourish your scalp, and leave hair looking fresh.

MAKES 1 TREATMENT

½ cup water
2 tablespoons apple
   cider vinegar

4 drops rosemary
   essential oil

2 drops lemon
   essential oil

CONTINUED »

1. In a plastic squeeze bottle, combine the water, vinegar, and rosemary and lemon essential oils.

2. Just before use, place your index finger over the bottle's tip and shake well.

3. After shampooing, apply the entire treatment to your scalp. Do not rinse.

4. Gently squeeze any excess solution from your hair. Apply a little conditioner to the ends if needed.

5. Towel your hair dry afterward and style it as usual.

OILY HAIR

Witch Hazel Scalp Toner

Witch hazel is a stylist's secret weapon thanks to astringent compounds that cut through scalp oil effortlessly. Lavender essential oil leaves an intoxicating fragrance that helps you forget this is a treatment. Mix it up with other oils like tea tree, sage, lemon, or peppermint. If you find that your scalp is becoming too dry, use the treatment every other day or try one made with apple cider vinegar instead of witch hazel.

MAKES 4 OUNCES

½ **cup alcohol-free witch hazel hydrosol**

1 **teaspoon lavender essential oil**

1. In a plastic squeeze bottle, combine the witch hazel and lavender essential oil. Label and date the bottle.

2. Just before use, place your index finger over the bottle's tip and shake well.

3. After washing your hair, apply enough of the entire treatment to moisten your scalp. Do not rinse.

CONTINUED »

4. Gently squeeze any excess solution from your hair. Apply a little conditioner to the ends if needed.

5. Towel your hair dry afterward and style it as usual. Use daily.

6. Store in a cool, dark place for up to 1 month.

OILY SKIN

Oregano and Yarrow Face Mask

Oregano is antibacterial and antibiotic to help oily skin regain equilibrium. Yarrow is antiseptic, astringent, and anti-inflammatory, and the clay helps pull impurities and toxins from the skin.

MAKES 3 MASKS

1 tablespoon
  dried oregano
1 tablespoon
  dried yarrow
1 tablespoon kaolin clay

1. Combine the oregano, yarrow, and kaolin clay and store in an airtight container. Label and date the container and store it in a cool, dark place for up to 2 years.

2. To use, after washing gently with a mild soap, combine 1 tablespoon of the blend with a liquid of your choice. Some good examples would be vinegar, witch hazel, lemon juice and water (50/50), or tea.

3. Spread the mixture over your face, avoiding the eyes. After 15 minutes, wash off gently. Pat dry.

4. If you'd like to utilize the scrubby, exfoliating effects of the herbs, after letting the mask rest on your face for 5 or 10 minutes, lather up a washcloth and rub in circular motions until the skin feels enlivened and slightly tingly. Do not do this if your skin feels irritated.

CONTINUED »

5. Use the mask once or twice a week. (I'm warning you: After this treatment, you may want to order a pizza.)

Herbal Mouthwash

Mouthwash can contain a lot of chemicals that aren't needed to help freshen your breath. This mouthwash is simple to make and works great. Once you get the general idea of how to make it, you can experiment with all sorts of flavors.

MAKES 16 OUNCES (ABOUT 122 RINSES)

2 cups chopped
  fresh peppermint
1½ cups grain alcohol
½ cup water

1. Follow the instructions in chapter 3 for making an alcohol tincture (page 32) using the peppermint and grain alcohol.

2. Once the tincture is ready, strain the peppermint, reserving the liquid, and pour the tincture into a 16-ounce glass bottle. Compost the solids.

3. Tighten the lid on the bottle and label with the name of the remedy and the instructions for use.

4. Put 1 to 2 dropperfuls (25 to 50 drops) of the tincture into a shot glass, and fill about three-quarters with water. Swish in the mouth like normal mouthwash. Do not swallow.

5. Store the bottle in a cool, dark location, where it will last indefinitely.

Aloe Vera and Tea Tree Oil Paste

The gel that contains the healing compounds of aloe vera includes essential amino acids, antioxidants, fatty acids, and minerals. It's also antimicrobial, antiviral, antifungal, and antibacterial. Adding tea tree oil to aloe vera makes it an even more potent remedy.

MAKES ABOUT ¾ CUP

1 (2-foot) fresh aloe leaf, or ½ cup alcohol-free aloe vera gel

¼ cup coconut oil

10 drops tea tree essential oil

1. Use a small knife to carefully slice open the aloe leaf. Scoop the clear gel out with a spoon and put it in a blender. Add the coconut oil. Blend for 30 to 60 seconds, until smooth.

2. Pour the mixture into an airtight glass container. Stir in the tea tree oil. Label and date the container.

3. Scoop out about 1 tablespoon of the paste and apply it to your skin. Use more if needed. Let it sit for 20 minutes and rinse with water and mild soap. If you use it on your scalp, wash it off with a mild shampoo.

4. Store the remainder of the paste in the refrigerator, and use within 1 week.

Calming Calendula Oil

A small bottle of calendula essential oil contains the medicinal components of thousands of calendula flowers, making it much more powerful than dried or fresh calendula. The wheat germ oil in this blend nourishes and soothes irritated skin, easing itching while promoting healing. Take 300 mg of milk thistle extract 3 times a day while using this treatment for even faster healing.

MAKES 25 DOSES

½ cup wheat germ oil
6 drops calendula
   essential oil
300 mg milk thistle
   extract (optional)

1. In a dark-colored glass bottle, combine the wheat germ oil and calendula essential oil. Cap the bottle tightly and shake well to combine. Label, date, and store in a cool, dark place. This treatment will keep for up to 1 year.

2. Apply the mixture to the affected areas at least twice a day for best results.

Chai Tonic Tea

Herbal teas like this chai, when taken regularly, are one of the best ways to relieve inflammation. Combine a diet rich in anti-inflammatory foods with a nourishing cup of chai. Consider drinking this chai as a tonic—a preparation of herbs that supports health and well-being.

MAKES 1 SERVING

1 cup coconut milk
1 teaspoon
   ground turmeric

½ teaspoon
   ground cinnamon
¼ teaspoon
   ground ginger

Pinch freshly ground
   pink pepper
½ teaspoon coconut oil

CONTINUED »

¼ teaspoon vanilla
  extract
½ to 1 teaspoon
  raw honey

1. In a small pot, heat the coconut milk over low heat. Add the turmeric, cinnamon, ginger, pepper, coconut oil, and vanilla. Simmer for 20 minutes, being careful not to bring the liquid to a boil.

2. Pour into a mug, and strain out the spices if you prefer.

3. Add honey to taste.

PUFFY EYES

Bright Eyes Compress

Disturbed sleep, too much screen time, and crying can make your eyes feel sore, tired, and swollen. Just 15 minutes with this compress will help your eyes feel brighter and look better. It may even improve your overall outlook.

**MAKES ENOUGH FOR
1 APPLICATION**

**2 tea bags (mint,
  chamomile,
  or echinacea)**

1. Brew a strong cup of tea using your choice of tea bags.

2. Cool the tea bags and place one on each eye. Rest them there for 15 minutes or so. Meanwhile, relax and meditate or listen to soothing or upbeat music. If you fall asleep, the tea bags won't hurt anything if they fall off.

3. Discard or compost the tea bags when you are through with them.

PUFFY EYES

Cool Chamomile Toner

This chamomile–witch hazel combo creates an amazing astringent that tightens tissue, reduces swelling, and eases inflammation. It isn't necessary to refrigerate this toner, but using it cold shrinks swelling more than applying the toner at room temperature.

MAKES ABOUT 2 OUNCES

¼ cup alcohol-free witch hazel hydrosol

4 drops chamomile essential oil

1. In a dark-colored glass bottle, combine the witch hazel with the chamomile essential oil. Shake well before each use. Label and date the bottle. Store in a cool, dark place for up to 1 year.

2. Using a cotton ball, apply 2 to 3 drops of toner to the area under each eye.

3. If you have a little time, lie back and rest for 5 to 10 minutes after application, placing a cloth under your eyes and topping the cloth with an ice cube beneath each eye.

PUFFY EYES

Lavender-Lemon Bedtime Serum

Let this magical de-puffer work while you sleep. Lavender and lemon essential oils help alleviate swollen under-eye tissue. Almond oil adds moisture, smoothing the appearance of delicate skin. Elevate your head with an extra pillow. Sleep on your back to help prevent fluid from accumulating in the tissue beneath your eyes.

MAKES ABOUT 2 OUNCES

¼ cup almond oil

10 drops lavender essential oil

10 drops lemon essential oil

CONTINUED »

1. In a dark-colored glass bottle, combine the almond oil, lavender essential oil, and lemon essential oil. Seal the bottle and shake well. Label and date the bottle.

2. Using your fingertips, gently dab 1 or 2 drops of serum under each eye.

3. Use nightly before bed. Store in a cool, dark place for up to 6 months.

PUFFY EYES

Rosemary Under-Eye Balm

Rosemary essential oil acts as a mild diuretic, which reduces under-eye swelling. It also contains anti-inflammatory compounds that help lighten discoloration, as well as nutrients that bolster compromised capillaries. If you plan to wear makeup, allow a few minutes for the balm to absorb before applying.

MAKES ABOUT 1 OUNCE

2 tablespoons argan oil
7 drops rosemary
   essential oil

1. In a dark-colored glass bottle, combine the argan oil and rosemary essential oil. Seal the bottle and shake well to combine. Label and date the bottle. Store in a cool, dark place for up to 6 months.

2. Using your fingertips, apply 1 to 2 drops to the under-eye area.

3. This treatment is suitable for daily use and can be applied morning and night.

SAFETY TIP: Do not allow the balm to enter the eyes.

Charcoal Purifying Mask

The ingredients of the dry mix work together to draw impurities from the skin and clear your pores. After a long day of perspiration, city exhaust, or any of the myriad assaults on our skin, this is excellent.

MAKES 3 TREATMENTS

1 tablespoon
activated charcoal

1 tablespoon kaolin or
green clay

1 tablespoon powdered
plantain leaf

1 to 2 tablespoons
liquid (yogurt, pureed
cucumber, hydrosols,
milk, or water)

1. In a small bowl, combine the charcoal, clay, and plantain leaf powder and mix very well.

2. Mix 1 tablespoon of the powder with 1 tablespoon of liquid, adding a teaspoon or so more as needed to make it spreadable.

3. Slather your face and neck, avoiding the eye area.

4. Relax for 15 minutes, and then remove gently with a washcloth and tepid water. Finish with a toner or moisturizer.

5. Store the dry powder in an airtight container in a cool, dark place for up to 2 years.

Hyssop Deep-Cleansing Mask

The ingredients of this mask clean and freshen the skin while drawing impurities from the pores. It's good for any skin type and can be adjusted to be more astringent or more emollient by changing the liquid used. Oil or yogurt might be used for drier skin types, whereas witch hazel or black tea would act as astringents for more oily skin.

CONTINUED »

**MAKES ABOUT
5 MASK APPLICATIONS**

2 tablespoons
dried hyssop

2 teaspoons
dried plantain

2 tablespoons ground
kaolin or French
green clay

2 teaspoons ground
activated charcoal

1. In a blender or coffee grinder, or using a mortar and pestle, grind the hyssop and plantain to a fine powder.

2. Transfer the powder to a small bowl and mix in the kaolin and activated charcoal. Place in a small jar, seal, label, date, and store in a cool, dark place until ready to use. It will last for up to 2 years.

3. To use, choose your preferred base or liquid—you can use plain water, oil, rose water, plain yogurt, witch hazel, carrot or cucumber juice, or milk. (Anything liquid will work, as long as it is skin-safe.) Mix 1 tablespoon of the powder mixture with enough of the base or liquid to make a thin, spreadable paste (the amount of base and liquid will vary greatly depending on what you use, but start with 1 teaspoon of liquid and keep adding until the desired consistency is reached).

4. Spread the mask on your face, relax for 10 or 15 minutes, and then rinse it off.

RESIDUE AND CLOGGED PORES

Lavender Bath Bombs

Lavender essential oil is very relaxing, and it's safe for kids. Other scents can be substituted, such as tangerine, chamomile, and rose geranium.

**MAKES 4 TO 6 BATH BOMBS,
DEPENDING ON SIZE**

1 cup baking soda
1 cup citric acid

½ cup cornstarch
5 drops red food
coloring (optional)

5 drops blue food
coloring (optional)
3 tablespoons olive oil

CONTINUED »

1½ teaspoons water

1½ dropperfuls (about 38 drops) lavender essential oil

1. In a medium bowl, combine the baking soda, citric acid, and cornstarch. Add the food colorings (if using), drop by drop, and stir well to distribute. Add the oils and water slowly, drop by drop, to the bowl of dry ingredients, mixing constantly. Alternatively, use a sprayer bottle, spray a couple times, mix well, spray, mix, and so on. Adding the liquid ingredients too quickly will cause the mixture to fizz.

2. The mixture should eventually clump together like damp sand. Either squeeze very tightly into balls with your hands, or pack well into molds.

3. Allow to dry for 24 hours. If the bath bombs won't pop out of the molds, freeze them briefly, then try again.

4. Plop one into the bath to soften the water and make it smell great.

5. Keep the bath bombs in a labeled, airtight container. Use within 6 months.

RESIDUE AND CLOGGED PORES

Soap Stones

These soaps provide some serious scrubbing while the tea tree and lavender essential oils add their antibiotic, antibacterial, and antifungal properties. They smell good, too!

CONTINUED »

MAKES 8 (4-OUNCE) BARS

24 ounces melt and
    pour (glycerin)
    soap base
8 ounces pumice
    powder
½ teaspoon tea tree
    essential oil
½ teaspoon lavender
    essential oil

1. Chop the soap base into chunks. The smaller the chunks, the more easily they will melt. The soap can be melted using a double boiler, or you can use a microwave, heating 30 or 60 seconds at a time.

2. When the soap is about 80 percent melted, stop heating and stir until it is all melted. Quickly stir in the pumice and tea tree and lavender essential oils. The cooler pumice will speed hardening. If necessary, heat the mixture for an additional 30 seconds.

3. Pour the liquid into molds. Allow time to set up. It will take up to 1 hour at room temperature, or you can put the soaps in the refrigerator to cut that setting time in half. If you don't have molds, lined muffin tins are nice, or you can just use a glass 8-by-8-inch pan and cut the soap into 9 squares.

4. Use like any bar soap, and keep it out of pooled water between uses so it lasts longer.

5. Wrap the bars in plastic wrap. Melt and pour soap bases are humectant and will draw moisture from the air if left unwrapped. Label and date the wrapped soaps.

ROSACEA

Gentle Chamomile Facial Toner

With terpene bisabolol, a natural pain and inflammation reliever, chamomile balances troubled skin, easing discomfort and redness. Make a new batch of this toner every few days so you always have some on hand.

CONTINUED »

MAKES ABOUT ½ CUP

1 cup water
1 handful dried
  chamomile flowers,
  or 3 handfuls fresh
  chamomile flowers

1. In a small saucepan, combine the water and chamomile and bring to a boil over high heat. Reduce the heat to low and simmer for 15 minutes or until the liquid reduces by half.

2. Let the liquid cool completely, and strain it into a glass jar. Compost the solids. Label and date the jar.

3. To apply the solution, soak a cotton ball and spread a thin layer over your freshly washed face. Let the toner dry naturally before applying your favorite moisturizer.

4. Use once or twice daily.

5. Store in the refrigerator for up to 3 days.

ROSACEA

Lavender–Aloe Vera Moisturizer

Lavender and aloe vera make an extremely effective healing duo with their natural antiseptic, anti-inflammatory, and soothing powers. Keep this moisturizer refrigerated if you use fresh aloe vera gel rather than the pre-packaged kind.

MAKES ABOUT 1 OUNCE

2 tablespoons
  alcohol-free aloe
  vera gel
8 drops lavender
  essential oil

1. In a small bowl, whisk together the aloe vera gel and lavender essential oil until thoroughly blended.

2. Transfer the moisturizer to a glass jar with a tight-fitting lid. Label and date the jar.

3. Using your fingertips, apply a thin layer of moisturizer to your face, neck, and chest. Let it absorb completely before applying any other products.

4. Use once or twice daily and within 2 years.

All-Purpose Calendula Salve

This salve comes in handy all year. From small boo-boos and skeeter bites to burns, cuts, chapped hands, and bruises, it soothes everything. I like to use it on days I forget to put moisturizer on my face, too.

MAKES 8 TO 10 OUNCES

1 cup fresh calendula
   flowers, or ½ cup dried
1½ cups olive oil
1 to 1½ ounces beeswax
20 drops lavender
   essential oil (optional)
20 drops tea tree
   essential oil (optional)

1. Use whatever method you prefer to infuse the calendula into the oil (page 30).

2. Strain the liquid into a small saucepan, squeezing as much oil from the flowers as possible. The goal is to have at least 1 cup of oil. Compost the solids.

3. Gently heat the oil with the beeswax over medium-low heat until the wax is liquefied. Stir the mixture well to be sure all the wax is incorporated. If including the essential oils, add them to the mixture.

4. Pour the salve into jars. When it has hardened and cooled, place lids on the jars, label, and date them.

5. To use, apply a thin layer of salve to the skin and gently massage it in.

6. Store in a cool, dark place for up to 1 year.

Aloe, Comfrey, and Lavender Soap

This soap is especially soothing. It can be used for all kinds of inflamed or reddened skin conditions, as well as burns, stings, and irritations.

CONTINUED »

The additions to the soap have long been used for skin conditions. Aloe and lavender are both exceptional for any kind of burn, while the allantoin in comfrey heals skin quickly.

MAKES 9 (4-OUNCE) BARS, DEPENDING ON SIZE OF MOLDS

1 pound melt and pour (glycerin) soap base
¼ cup alcohol-free aloe vera gel
2 ounces strong comfrey tea
30 drops lavender essential oil

1. Chop the soap base into chunks. The smaller the chunks, the more easily they will melt.

2. In a double boiler, melt the soap over medium heat.

3. When the soap is about 80 percent liquid, stop heating and stir until it is all melted. Quickly add the aloe vera gel, comfrey tea, and lavender essential oil. If necessary, heat for an additional 30 seconds.

4. Pour into molds. Allow time to set up. It takes up to an hour at room temperature, or you can put the soaps in the refrigerator to cut that in half. If you don't have molds, lined muffin tins are nice, or you can just use a glass 8-by-8-inch pan and cut into 9 squares.

5. Use as any other bar soap. Wrap, label, date, and keep dry between uses.

SKIN CONDITIONS

Boo-Boo Balm

It is always good to have a nice salve handy for all kinds of skin issues, from rashes to splinters to bumps and bruises. This is a nice one. If you'd like to make this with fresh herbs, triple the herb amounts listed.

MAKES ABOUT 6 OUNCES

1 cup olive oil

1 tablespoon dried plantain leaf

1 tablespoon dried calendula

CONTINUED »

1 tablespoon
  dried comfrey
1 tablespoon
  dried chickweed
1 tablespoon dried
  burdock leaf
½ to 1 ounce beeswax

1. In a double boiler, combine the olive oil, plantain, calendula, comfrey, chickweed, and burdock and heat to a simmer over medium-low heat.

2. Remove from the heat, then heat again 1 or 2 times. Cool and allow to steep overnight.

3. The herbs will absorb a lot of the oil. Strain into a small jar and squeeze the herbs to get every bit of the oil that you can. Compost the solids.

4. Measure the oil. If it is 1 cup, you'll use 1 ounce of beeswax. For ¾ cup, you'll need ¾ ounce of beeswax. If it is ½ cup, it will be ½ ounce of beeswax. The amount of beeswax will determine how hard or loose the salve is.

5. Combine the oil and beeswax and heat gently until the wax is melted. Pour into jars or tins, label, and date.

6. Apply liberally to irritated skin, stings, rashes, and dry, itchy patches.

7. Salves have a good shelf life. It should last several months if not exposed to extreme heat. To avoid molding, do not introduce moisture to the salve.

SKIN CONDITIONS

Calendula Sunshine Bath Soak

This is a rejuvenating and soothing bath that feels incredible after too much time in the sun or garden. The magnesium in Epsom salts is great for overworked muscles. With the addition of some other ingredients, you'll step out of

CONTINUED »

the bath a new person. The scents and healing properties of the herbs and the pure relaxation of a warm bath combine to heal scratches, bug bites, windburn, or sunburn.

MAKES 12 BATH SOAKS

1 cup dried calendula
  flowers, chopped
1 cup dried comfrey leaf
½ cup dried yarrow
¼ cup dried elderflower
3 tablespoons dried
  lavender flowers
20 drops lemon
  essential oil
3 cups Epsom salts

1. In a medium bowl, combine the calendula, comfrey, yarrow, elderflower, and lavender.

2. In a separate bowl, combine the lemon essential oil and Epsom salts and mix.

3. Combine both mixtures into a 2-quart jar, label with the date, and store in a cool, dark place for up to 1 year. If you're keeping it near the tub, a (recycled) plastic jar is safest.

4. To use, place ½ cup of the soak in a muslin bag or into a washcloth and tie securely. Heat a quart of water on the stove and steep the bath soak in it for 10 to 15 minutes.

5. Pour the hot liquid into the bath. Soak.

SKIN CONDITIONS

Facial Steam

Herbal steams are helpful in several ways. The steam opens pores and loosens blackheads and dead skin. Herbal properties in the steam (like weak hydrosols) carry many benefits, and they are deposited directly onto the skin and through the respiratory system. There are many herbs that can be used in steams, for various skin issues. Use this recipe as a jumping-off point to relieve clogged pores, dull skin, and aching sinuses.

MAKES 1 TREATMENT

1 to 2 quarts water

¾ cup dried
  chamomile flowers

¼ cup dried
  lavender flowers

CONTINUED »

1. In a large saucepan, bring the water to a boil over high heat.

2. Place the herbs in a wide heatproof bowl. Pour the boiling water over the herbs, allowing them to steep for a few minutes while the water cools slightly.

3. Sit in a chair with your face over the bowl. Drape a towel over the back of your head and neck and let it fall down around the outside of the bowl, making a tent to trap the steam.

4. Spend 10 to 15 minutes enjoying the vapors.

5. Apply a moisturizer.

SKIN CONDITIONS

Rose Splash

This remedy can be used to wake up and brighten dull skin. I use rose in this, but there can be many herbs substituted, depending on preference. Lavender, sage, holy basil, bay leaves ... anything that you'd like to try!

MAKES 12 OUNCES

2 cups dried rose petals
¾ cup water
1 cup apple cider vinegar
2 teaspoons raw honey

1. In a large saucepan, combine the rose petals and water and bring the mixture to a boil over medium-high heat. Remove the pan from the heat and let steep for 1 hour.

2. Heat over medium-low heat, just to a simmer one more time, then remove the pan from the heat and let the mixture steep for 1 hour more. Strain the liquid into a jar and mix in the vinegar and honey. Compost the solids. Label and date the jar.

CONTINUED »

3. Use cotton balls to apply the treatment directly to your skin, or simply pour a bit into the palm of your hand, splash it onto your face, and massage it in. It also makes a wonderful spray!

4. This splash is best kept refrigerated. Or, keep about ½ cup handy and refrigerate the rest. Use within a month. If you'd like it to last longer, add an ounce or two of vodka.

SKIN IRRITATION

Comfrey and Calendula Skin Soother

This skin soother is great for sunburn, windburn, rashes, and irritations of the skin. This can also be used on a brush-burn type of injury. Broken skin or wounds should be cleaned well before use. Comfrey is such a speedy healer that it has been known to regenerate healthy skin around dirt, causing possible future infection.

MAKES 6 OUNCES

¾ cup water

2 tablespoons dried comfrey leaf

2 tablespoons dried calendula blossoms

2 tablespoons 100-proof alcohol

1. In a small saucepan, bring the water to a boil over high heat.

2. Remove the pan from the heat. Add the comfrey and calendula and steep for 30 minutes.

3. Strain into a 1-cup glass measuring cup. The comfrey will retain a good bit of the liquid, but give it a squeeze to get as close to ⅝ cup of water as possible. Compost the solids.

4. Let cool completely, then add the alcohol. Transfer to a small jar or spray bottle. Label and date the jar or bottle.

5. Use within a week, or refrigerate for 2 weeks.

Day-to-Night Liniment

You need to change from work clothes into evening wear, and your skin and general energy level aren't keeping up with the changes? This might be just what you need. The ingredients are energizing physically and emotionally, with the added benefit of soothing the aches and pains of the day. In addition to the bright fragrances, this liniment is analgesic and anti-inflammatory. The ginger warms, increasing circulation, the clove mildly numbs (in case you were on your feet all day), and the mint cools. It's a great combination!

MAKES 2 CUPS

¼ **cup grated**
fresh ginger
2 **cups vodka**
15 **drops peppermint**
essential oil
15 **drops clove**
essential oil

1. In a jar, combine the ginger and vodka. Seal and let the mixture infuse for 2 weeks.

2. Strain the liquid into a separate jar and compost the solids. Add the peppermint oil and clove oil. Cover, label, and date the jar.

3. Massage into sore areas gently to relieve pain.

4. Store in a cool, dark place. This will keep for years.

Green Tea Astringent Toner

The antibacterial and anti-inflammatory aspects of green tea, combined with the astringency of witch hazel hydrosol, all conspire to minimize pores and clear up blemishes and irritation. This toner is also excellent for use after wearing a mask over the nose and mouth. It can also be used as an unscented aftershave.

CONTINUED »

MAKES 4 OUNCES

¼ cup water

1 tablespoon green
   tea leaves

¼ cup alcohol-free witch
   hazel hydrosol

1. In a small saucepan, bring the water to a boil over high heat. Steep the tea in the water for 30 minutes until it is quite strong.

2. Strain the liquid into a 1-cup glass measuring cup and compost the solids. Allow the tea to cool.

3. Combine the cooled tea with the witch hazel in a bottle that holds at least ½ cup. Label and date the bottle.

4. Keep the toner in the refrigerator and apply with a cotton ball for a refreshing, enlivening wake-up for your face.

5. Store at room temperature for up to 1 week or in the refrigerator for 2 to 4 weeks. If you'd like it to last longer, add ½ ounce of rubbing alcohol or 100-proof alcohol (like vodka).

SKIN IRRITATION

Lavender Powder

This powder has several benefits. Lavender is soothing to the skin, so there's the comfort factor. It is also calming and relaxing, and helps slow down perspiration that comes from stress. It can help decrease fungal or bacterial issues forming from damp areas and creases. On top of all of this, it smells pleasant. You can increase the fragrance by adding 10 to 15 drops of lavender essential oils to the powder if desired.

MAKES 2 CUPS

1 cup arrowroot powder

½ cup cornstarch

¼ cup kaolin or French
   green clay

¼ cup dried lavender
   flowers, powdered
   in a blender or
   coffee grinder

CONTINUED »

1. In a 1-quart jar, combine the arrowroot, cornstarch, kaolin or French green clay, and lavender. Secure the lid and shake well. Keep the mix in the jar for at least 2 weeks or up to a month for the scent to permeate the other powders, shaking it at least once every few days. Label and date the jar. Store in a cool, dry place out of direct sunlight for up to 1 year.

2. To use, pour a small amount of the powder into the palm of your hand and smooth onto your body to remedy chafing or excessive perspiration.

SKIN IRRITATION

Refreshing Body Splash

Splash this on after a shower for a refreshing, nourishing treatment for your skin.

MAKES 16 OUNCES

1 cup boiling water

2 tablespoons dried basil

½ cup peppermint tincture

½ cup aloe vera juice

1. In a small bowl, combine the water and basil and steep for 20 minutes.

2. Strain into another small bowl. Compost the solids.

3. Add the tincture and aloe vera juice. Mix well.

4. Transfer to a 16-ounce glass bottle. Label and date the solution.

5. Shake the bottle, then pour some into your hand to splash onto your body. Alternatively, use a spray bottle to spray it on your body.

6. Store in the bathroom for quick access or in the refrigerator for a cooler splash, where it will last for up to 1 year. Unrefrigerated, this can last up to 6 months.

Rosy Milk Bath

Comfrey releases a mucilaginous yet luxurious property into the water, similar to oatmeal's silky, soothing benefits. Milk in baths has been revered for centuries, per-haps because of the fat content, which gives us the same benefits as oils without the slippery tub. Rose petals are a wonderful emollient. Together, these additions to the bath remove the discomfort from too much sun, wind, or not enough moisture.

MAKES 14 OR 15 BATHS

2 cups dried rose petals

2 cups dried comfrey

2 cups milk powder

½ cup old-fashioned rolled oats

1 to 2 quarts water

1. In a large bowl, combine rose, comfrey, milk powder, and oats. (If preferred, skip the powdered milk and add 1 to 2 quarts fresh milk directly to the bath, omitting the water.)

2. Put ½ cup of the mixture in a muslin bag. In a large saucepan, heat the water or fresh milk to boiling and steep the bag in the water or milk while running the bath.

3. Pour the water or milk and bag into the bathtub. Soak for 15 minutes or so.

4. Keep the leftover dry mixture in an airtight container, and label and date it accordingly. It will last for up to 1 year.

SKIN IRRITATION

Sunburn Soother Spray

Prevention is the best medicine, so when you're heading into the sun, be sure to cover up with a thin layer of clothing and a hat! For those times when you forget to do that, this spray helps soothe sunburns, ease the pain from them, and assist in healing the skin. This spray can be used on other burns as well.

CONTINUED »

MAKES 4 OUNCES

½ ounce mullein
   leaf tincture
½ ounce lavender
   tincture
½ ounce raspberry
   leaf–infused vinegar
½ ounce rose
   petal–infused vinegar
¼ cup water

1. In a 1-cup glass measuring cup, combine the mullein leaf tincture, lavender tincture, raspberry leaf–infused vinegar, rose petal–infused vinegar, and water and mix well.

2. Pour the tincture blend into a 4-ounce glass bottle with a spray-top lid.

3. Tighten the lid on the bottle. Label and date the spray.

4. Spray on sunburn for relief. Reapply as needed.

5. Store the bottle in a cool, dark location, where it will last indefinitely.

SKIN IRRITATION

Tea, Chamomile, and Rose Apres Sun Bath

Tea is anti-inflammatory, and chamomile has great healing properties for the skin. Rose cools and soothes. This combination works very well together for sunburn, windburn, or when your skin isn't "fitting right."

MAKES 1 BATH

1 cup water
1 heaping tablespoon
   black tea leaves,
   or 1 large
   (family-size) tea bag
¼ cup dried rose petals
¼ cup dried
   chamomile flowers
1 cup apple cider vinegar

1. In a small saucepan, bring the water to a boil over high heat.

2. Remove the pan from the heat. Add the tea, rose petals, and chamomile and allow to steep for 15 minutes.

3. Strain the liquid into a jar and compost the solids. Allow the liquid to cool, then add the vinegar.

4. Run a tepid bath and add the liquid. Climb in and be sure the affected area is submerged. Soak for

CONTINUED »

at least 15 minutes. For a sunburn, you want to remove the heat from the skin, so try to soak until the skin has cooled.

5. If a bath isn't feasible, this liquid can be cooled and used as a compress. It can also be used as a spray for large areas.

6. If used as a spray, keep in the refrigerator for up to a month in a labeled and dated bottle.

SORE FEET

"Oh, My Dogs Are Barking" Footbath

When our feet hurt, we really do hurt all over. It seems that the most stressful times in my life also involve dressy shoes that are never broken in or comfortable. Soaking your feet in warm, very strong herbal infusions can relax and enliven them, get the blood and possible swelling moving, soften callouses, and clean any developing blisters.

MAKES 1 SOAK

1 tablespoon dried
  lavender flowers
1 tablespoon dried sage
1 teaspoon dried
  rosemary
1 teaspoon dried
  monarda or oregano

1. Place the lavender, sage, rosemary, and monarda or oregano in a muslin or cotton bag, tie it closed, and lower it into a large pot filled with water. Cover the pot and simmer over low heat for 10 minutes.

2. Pour the liquid into a large heatproof basin, and adjust the temperature with cold water, adding a little at a time, until it is just right. The goal is for the water to be as hot as you can stand it without causing pain or discomfort. Be sure to have a towel nearby for when you finish.

CONTINUED »

3. Immerse your feet and relax. It's nice to have a teakettle with more hot water nearby to keep the soak going longer.

4. Discard the water after use.

SORE FEET

Tired Tootsies Soaking Tea

A plain mint tea is a wonderful, cooling foot soak after one of those days when you've been on your feet all day and they feel as if they may be on fire. Adding a few other ingredients makes it superb. The peppermint will cool. The comfrey will soothe. The lavender will help relax you. The vinegar will help slough off dead skin as you rub your feet on marbles or coarse salt. Finally, the oil will moisturize.

MAKES 1 TREATMENT

1 cup apple
   cider vinegar
2 cups water
3 tablespoons
   dried peppermint
2 tablespoons dried
   comfrey leaf
2 tablespoons dried
   lavender flowers
1 tablespoon olive oil
Marbles or
   coarse salt, for
   sloughing (optional)

1. In a medium saucepan, bring the vinegar and water to a boil over medium heat.

2. Remove the pan from the heat. Add the peppermint, comfrey, and lavender and let steep for 10 minutes.

3. Strain into a heatproof basin of warm water. Compost the solids. Add the olive oil to the basin.

4. Sit back, soak your feet, enjoy a nice cup of tea, and relax for 15 minutes while your feet recover.

5. Add marbles or salt (if using). Place your feet in the basin and massage them on the salt or marbles.

Lavender–Witch Hazel Spritz

Witch hazel tones and tightens skin, while lavender helps alleviate pain and inflammation.

MAKES ABOUT 8 OUNCES

1 (8-ounce) bottle
  alcohol-free witch
  hazel hydrosol
32 drops lavender
  essential oil

1. In a glass bottle, combine the witch hazel and lavender essential oil.

2. Cap tightly, then shake well. Label and date the bottle.

3. Spray onto your legs each morning and evening, massaging lightly afterward.

4. Use as often as needed to keep your legs feeling comfortable. Store in a cool, dark place between uses, and use within 1 month.

Soothing Witch Hazel Liniment

Soothe the discomfort of varicose veins with this lightweight witch hazel liniment. Over time, this liniment may also help shrink swollen leg tissue and reduce the appearance of varicose veins.

MAKES 50 DOSES

1 cup alcohol
  (40-percent or higher)
1 cup alcohol-free witch
  hazel hydrosol

1. In a dark-colored glass bottle with a narrow neck, combine the alcohol and witch hazel. Label and date the bottle.

2. Apply the liniment generously with a cotton pad twice a day, shaking the bottle well before each use. After the liniment dries, use your favorite lotion to keep skin feeling soft and supple.

3. Store it in a cool, dark place. This liniment will last indefinitely when properly stored.

Geranium-Honey Hair Repair

With honey and olive oil to moisturize, this nourishing treatment also contains geranium essential oil to strengthen hair. Use between haircuts to fortify strands and preserve that healthy, freshly cut salon look.

MAKES 1 TREATMENT

1 tablespoon olive oil
1 tablespoon raw honey
3 drops geranium
  essential oil

1. In a small microwave-safe bowl, combine the olive oil and honey. Microwave on low power for 15 seconds. Stir the honey and olive oil together. If the honey is still too thick to stir into the olive oil, microwave for another 15 seconds and stir again.

2. Stir in the geranium essential oil.

3. Dampen your hair and apply the entire treatment.

4. Cover your head with a disposable shower cap, then wrap it with a towel.

5. Leave the hair repair in place for 10 to 15 minutes, then wash, condition, and style as usual.

6. Repeat once or twice weekly.

Soothing Stretch Mark Butter

Whether you're trying to prevent new stretch marks from forming or are hoping to help old ones fade, this nourishing butter will help. Keeping skin moisturized aids healing and prevents damage.

CONTINUED »

MAKES 50 DOSES

1 cup cocoa butter
4 tablespoons finely
    grated beeswax
40 drops lavender
    essential oil

1. In a medium saucepan, warm the cocoa butter and beeswax over low to medium-low heat, warming the mixture just until the beeswax melts. Remove the saucepan from the heat, then stir in the lavender essential oil.

2. Pour the mixture into a wide-mouth jar or tin and allow it to cool completely before capping. Label and date the jar.

3. Use a generous amount of the butter on stretch marks (or where new stretch marks may form) at least twice a day.

4. Store it in a cool, dark place for up to 1 year.

WARTS

Natural Garlic Wart Remover

If you are suffering from warts, there's no need to purchase an expensive chemical treatment to remove them. This simple two-ingredient wart remover is completely natural and is wonderfully effective. Although it often works the first time, you may need to reapply it a few times to remove the wart completely.

MAKES 1 DOSE

1 garlic clove
1 vitamin E capsule, any
    size (or an all-purpose
    salve, since it is just
    protecting the skin
    around the wart)

1. Smash and peel the garlic clove.

2. Pierce the vitamin E capsule and apply it to the skin surrounding the wart but not to the wart itself. Place the garlic clove over the wart and cover it with an adhesive bandage.

CONTINUED »

3. Leave the bandage in place for 24 hours. When you remove the bandage, you should see a blister. Don't disturb it—within about 1 week, your wart should fall off. Repeat the treatment the following week if the wart hasn't come off. If no change has occurred after two treatments, see your doctor or dermatologist for wart removal.

WRINKLES

Frankincense-Lavender Skin Serum

This light herbal serum offers a powerhouse of age-defying oils. Macadamia rejuvenates tired, aging skin. Lavender calms and moisturizes. Meadowfoam delivers major antioxidants. And frankincense balances pH while repairing skin cells.

MAKES 2 OUNCES

2 tablespoons
  macadamia nut oil
1½ tablespoons
  meadowfoam seed oil
15 drops frankincense
  (boswellia)
  essential oil
10 drops lavender
  essential oil

1. In a dark-colored glass bottle fitted with a glass dropper, combine the macadamia, meadowfoam, frankincense (boswellia), and lavender essential oils. Cover and shake for 30 seconds to blend. Label and date the bottle.

2. With your fingertips, apply a thin layer to your skin, focusing on crow's feet and laugh lines. Let the serum absorb into your skin. Follow up with your favorite moisturizer.

3. You can use this serum to hydrate your entire face, if you like.

4. Store it in a cool, dark place for up to 6 months.

Lavender Toner with Vitamins C and E

This fragrant toner nourishes skin and provides a lightweight layer of protective moisture. With daily use, it reduces the appearance of crow's feet and dry, indoor-air-damaged skin.

MAKES 2 OUNCES

3½ tablespoons rose hydrosol

¾ teaspoon vitamin C crystals

20 drops lavender essential oil

20 drops vitamin E oil

1. In a small bowl, combine the rose hydrosol and vitamin C crystals. Stir gently until the vitamin C crystals are dissolved.

2. Using a funnel, transfer the liquid to a dark-colored glass bottle. Carefully add the lavender essential oil and vitamin E oil to the bottle. Cover and shake well. Label and date the bottle.

3. Using a cotton ball, apply a few drops to your clean face. Follow up with your favorite moisturizer.

4. Use this toner each morning and night.

5. Store in a cool, dark place for up to 3 months.

Rosemary-Papaya Facial Mask

Ready to get your glow back? Fresh papaya contains vitamin C to stimulate collagen production, and papain, an enzyme that exfoliates and tightens pores. Rosemary essential oil speeds cell renewal and improves circulation.

CONTINUED »

MAKES 1 TREATMENT

¼ cup fresh
   papaya puree
6 drops rosemary
   essential oil

1. In a small bowl, combine the papaya and rosemary essential oil.

2. Using your fingertips, apply the mixture to your freshly washed face, focusing on crow's feet and laugh lines.

3. Relax for 15 minutes. If the mixture seems too slippery, keep it in place by covering your face with a paper or cotton facial mask.

4. When finished, rinse your face with cool water and apply your favorite moisturizer.

5. You may feel a tingling sensation while this mask is doing its work. If you experience discomfort, remove the treatment.

WRINKLES

Simply Bewitching Wrinkle Reducer

Witch hazel contains antioxidants that help prevent tissue breakdown, and argan oil helps keep skin hydrated and promotes elasticity. Although this treatment is a very simple one, it will leave your face glowing, and over time, you'll notice wrinkles beginning to fade.

MAKES 15 DOSES

2 tablespoons argan oil
2 tablespoons
   alcohol-free witch
   hazel hydrosol

1. In a dark-colored glass bottle with a narrow neck, combine the argan oil and witch hazel. Label and date the bottle.

2. Shake well and apply a small amount to a cotton ball or cotton pad, then apply the mixture to clean skin, focusing on areas with wrinkles, age spots, and spider veins.

3. Use the mixture twice a day as part of your regular skin-care regimen. Store in a cool, dark place. This treatment will keep for up to 2 months.

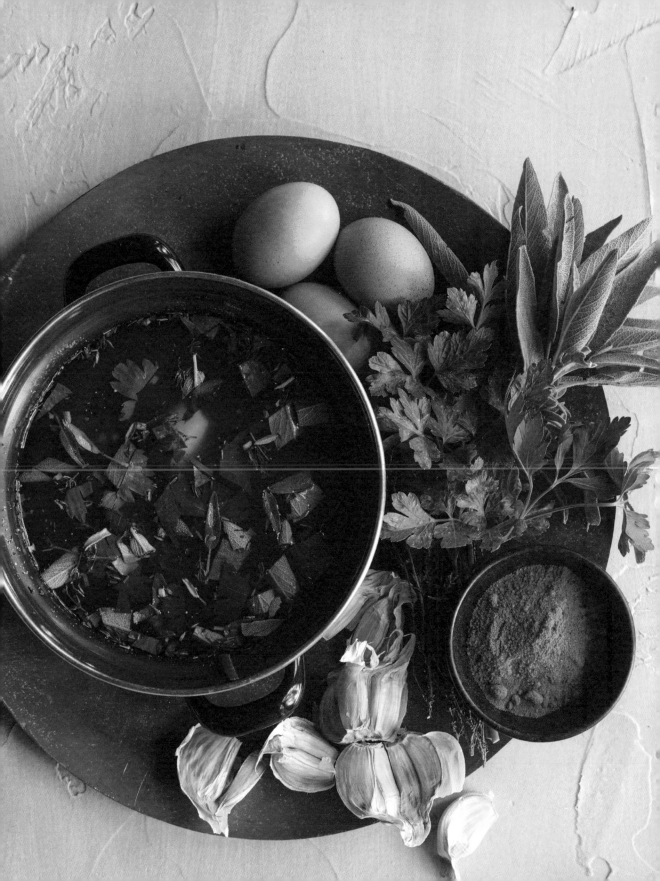

Measurement Conversions

VOLUME EQUIVALENTS

	U.S. STANDARD	U.S. STANDARD (OUNCES)	METRIC (APPROXIMATE)
LIQUID	2 tablespoons	1 fl. oz.	30 mL
	¼ cup	2 fl. oz.	60 mL
	½ cup	4 fl. oz.	120 mL
	1 cup	8 fl. oz.	240 mL
	1½ cups	12 fl. oz.	355 mL
	2 cups or 1 pint	16 fl. oz.	475 mL
	4 cups or 1 quart	32 fl. oz.	1 L
DRY	¼ teaspoon	–	1 mL
	½ teaspoon	–	2 mL
	¾ teaspoon	–	4 mL
	1 teaspoon	–	5 mL
	1 tablespoon	–	15 mL
	¼ cup	–	59 mL
	⅓ cup	–	79 mL
	½ cup	–	118 mL
	⅔ cup	–	156 mL
	¾ cup	–	177 mL
	1 cup	–	235 mL
	2 cups or 1 pint	–	475 mL
	3 cups	–	700 mL
	4 cups or 1 quart	–	1 L
	½ gallon	–	2 L
	1 gallon	–	4 L

OVEN TEMPERATURES

FAHRENHEIT	CELSIUS (APPROXIMATE)
300°F	150°C
325°F	165°C
350°F	180°C
375°F	190°C
400°F	200°C
425°F	220°C
450°F	230°C

WEIGHT EQUIVALENTS

1 ounce	30 g
2 ounces	60 g
4 ounces	115 g
8 ounces	225 g
12 ounces	340 g
16 ounces or 1 pound	455 g

Sourcing High-Quality Herbs and Supplies

There are a lot of excellent suppliers for all the things written about in this book, and here are some of my favorites that I have purchased from over the years. Many of them are owned by people I know. Personally, I prefer to work with businesses that are owned by people you can talk to directly. I do not purchase from multilevel essential oil companies, nor from businesses that claim to be the *only* real or good product, costing a fortune with no real benefit. It simply isn't true. There are many (most of them, really) good, honest suppliers. Most of these suppliers offer organic or fair-trade ingredients. You'll find seeds and plants, a copper still supplier, and lots of really fun ingredients! You may want to start clearing out the guest room now so you have a place for your own apothecary. (Don't say I didn't warn you!)

BRAMBLE BERRY
BrambleBerry.com (Washington)
Oils, butters, soap bases, molds, waxes, and essential oils

BULK APOTHECARY
BulkApothecary.com (Ohio)
Packaging, soap bases, essential oils, colors, and flavors

CANDLES AND SUPPLIES
CandlesAndSupplies.com (Pennsylvania)
Oils, butters, packaging and containers, waxes, essential oils, hydrosols, soap bases, and copper stills

iHERB
iHerb.com (California)
Retail website for herbs, essential oils, butters, waxes, implements, and more

MOUNTAIN ROSE HERBS

MountainRoseHerbs.com (Oregon)

Good-quality organic herbs and just about everything else

NATURE'S GIFT

NaturesGift.com (Tennessee)

High-quality essential oils and hydrosols

SEED SAVERS EXCHANGE

SeedSavers.org (Iowa)

Nonprofit dedicated to preserving organic, heirloom, and non-GMO seeds

SKS BOTTLES

SKS-Bottle.com (East Coast)

Bottles, jars, and tins

SPECIALTY BOTTLE

SpecialtyBottle.com (West Coast)

Bottles, jars, and tins

STRICTLY MEDICINAL SEEDS

StrictlyMedicinalSeeds.com (Oregon)

Seeds and plants of hundreds of medicinal herbs. Fabulous quality, always the correct species.

THE ESSENTIAL HERBAL

EssentialHerbal.com (Pennsylvania)

Incense supplies, tea implements, and single tinctures

THE ROSEMARY HOUSE

TheRosemaryHouse.com (Pennsylvania)

Wide variety of ingredients, teas, and tinctures

Resources

AMERICAN HERBALISTS GUILD

AmericanHerbalistsGuild.com

A website where you can find qualified herbalists who have passed stringent testing. Members can take online courses that are frequently offered, and there is an annual
conference.

CHESTNUT SCHOOL OF HERBAL MEDICINE

ChestnutHerbs.com

Led by Juliet Blankespoor, Chestnut has a beautiful, welcoming aesthetic and a wonderful blog that shares a huge amount of information.

***ESSENTIAL HERBAL* MAGAZINE**

EssentialHerbal.com

A website and magazine that covers all aspects of herbalism, including medicinal, culinary, decorative, gardening, and more. Owned and edited by yours truly.

HERBAL ROOTS ZINE

HerbalRootsZine.org

A unique magazine and membership website that teaches children and beginners through experience, story, song, and *fun*. HRz is the only herbal curriculum that uses all four learning styles (visual, auditory, reading, and kinesthetic) to fully immerse students in the herbal learning experience.

INTERNATIONAL HERB ASSOCIATION

iHerb.org

An organization of welcoming herbal professionals and people who would like to make herbs their profession. All aspects of herbalism included.

THE HERBAL ACADEMY

TheHerbalAcademy.com

A vast web of educators, writers, and illustrators combine to create the Academy, providing a selection of courses from beginner to professional.

LEARNING HERBS AND HERB MENTOR

LearningHerbs.com

A subscription-based online community that offers classes (additional fee) frequently and sends out a regular newsletter via email, typically including an interesting recipe.

SCIENCE & ART OF HERBALISM

ScienceAndArtOfHerbalism.com

The original correspondence course for herbalists, Rosemary Gladstar and her lovely staff present a useful and versatile group of courses.

UNITED PLANT SAVERS

UnitedPlantSavers.org

An organization providing information on the ethical harvesting of herbs. Before you head out into the woods with your basket and snippers, learn about the plants that are being overharvested or have lost their habitat.

Finally, please find your local herb shops and herb clubs/groups. Participate in festivals in your area and take classes in person whenever possible. It's fun to travel to conferences, but it's more valuable to encourage and help develop a local herbal community. If it isn't there, find people who would like to meet and learn together! Support local herbal businesses whenever possible.

References

"4 Ways to Feel Fantastic This Autumn." *Natural Health*. Accessed July 6, 2021. NaturalHealthWoman.com/4-ways-to-feel-fantastic-this-autumn.

Akhondzadeh, S., H. R. Naghavi, M. Vazirian, A. Shayeganpour, et al. "Passionflower in the Treatment of Generalized Anxiety: A Pilot Doubleblind Randomized Controlled Trial with Oxazepam." *Journal of Clinical Pharmacy and Therapeutics* 26, no. 5 (Oct 2001): 363–7. DOI:10.1046/j.1365-2710.2001.00367.x.

Ashpari, Zohra. "The Calming Effects of Passion-flower." Healthline. Last modified September 29, 2018. Healthline.com/health/anxiety/calming-effects-of-passionflower.

Brown, Kristine. *Herbalism at Home: 125 Recipes for Everyday Health*. Emeryville: Rockridge Press, 2019.

Brown, Kristine. *The Homesteader's Guide to Growing Herbs: Learn to Grow, Prepare, and Use Herbs*. Emeryville: Rockridge Press, 2020.

Do-It-Yourself Herbal Medicine: Home-Crafted Remedies for Health & Beauty. Berkeley: Sonoma Press, 2015.

Hess, Susan, and Tina Sams. *The Herbal Medicine Cookbook: Everyday Recipes to Boost Your Health*. Emeryville: Rockridge Press, 2019.

Home Remedies RX: DIY Prescriptions When You Need Them Most. Berkeley: Althea Press, 2014.

Lam, Kim. *The Holistic Health Handbook: Healing Remedies for Common Ailments*. Emeryville: Rockridge Press, 2020.

Movafegh, A., R. Alizadeh, F. Hajimohamadi, F. Esfehani, and M. Nejatfar. "Preoperative Oral Passiflora Incarnata Reduces Anxiety in Ambulatory Surgery Patients: A Double-Blind, Placebo-Controlled Study." *Anesthesia and Analgesia* 106, no. 6 (June 2008): 1728–1732. DOI:10.1213/ane.0b013e318172c3f9.

Panahi, Yunes, Mohsen Taghizadeh, Eisa Tahmasbpour Marzony, and Amirhossein Sahebkar. "Rosemary Oil vs. Minoxidil 2% for the Treatment of Androgenetic Alopecia: A Randomized Comparative Trial." *SKINmed* 13, no. 1 (2015): 15–21.

"Pennyroyal Oil." LiverTox. Last modified March 28, 2020. NCBI.NLM.NIH.gov /books/NBK548673/.

Rahbardar, Mahboobeh Ghasemzadeh, and Hossein Hosseinzadeh. "Therapeutic Effects of Rosemary (Rosemarinus officinalis L.) and Its Active Constituents on Nervous System Disorders." *Iranian Journal of Basic Medical Sciences* 23, no. 9 (September 2020): 1100–1112. DOI:10.22038/ijbms.2020.45269.10541.

Sams, Tina. *Herbal Medicine for Emotional Healing: 101 Natural Remedies for Anxiety, Depression, Sleep, and More*. Emeryville: Rockridge Press, 2020.

Sams, Tina. *The Healing Power of Herbs: Medicinal Herbs for Common Ailments*. Emeryville: Althea Press, 2019.

Srivastava, Janmejai K., Eswar Shankar, and Sanjay Gupta. "Chamomile: A Herbal Medicine of the Past with Bright Future." *Molecular Medicine Reports* 3, no. 6 (November 2010): 895–901. DOI:10.3892/mmr.2010.377.

The Practical Herbal Medicine Handbook: Your Quick Reference Guide to Healing Herbs & Remedies. Berkeley: Althea Press, 2014.

Herb Index

R

Y

Ailment Index

O

Oily hair
  Rosemary-Lemon Rinse, 345–346
  Witch Hazel Scalp Toner, 346–347
Oily skin
  Oregano and Yarrow Face
    Mask, 347–348
Oral hygiene
  Herbal Mouthwash, 348

P

Pain. *See* Aches and pains
Pinkeye
  Chamomile Compress, 217
Poison ivy
  Poison Ivy and Poison Oak
    Relief, 217–218
  Witch Hazel Compress, 218
Premenstrual syndrome (PMS)
  Balance Tea Blend, 219
  Ginger–Black Cohosh Tonic, 219–220
Psoriasis
  Aloe Vera and Tea Tree Oil Paste, 349
  Calming Calendula Oil, 350
  Chai Tonic Tea, 350–351
Puffy eyes
  Bright Eyes Compress, 351
  Cool Chamomile Toner, 352
  Lavender-Lemon Bedtime
    Serum, 352–353
  Rosemary Under-Eye Balm, 353

R

Residue and clogged pores
  Charcoal Purifying Mask, 354
  Hyssop Deep-Cleansing Mask, 354–355
  Lavender Bath Bombs, 355–356
  Soap Stones, 356–357
Respiratory illness. *See also* Coughs
  Echinacea Elderberry
    Gummies, 220–221

  Marseilles Vinegar, 221–222
  Sage and Garlic Soup, 222–223
Restlessness. *See also* Sleep issues
  Lavender Bath Bombs, 355–356
  Perchance to Dream Pillow, 286–287
  Sweet Dreams Elixir, 287
Ringworm
  Lavender–Tea Tree Toner, 223
  Ringworm Relief, 224
Rosacea
  Gentle Chamomile Facial
    Toner, 357–358
  Lavender–Aloe Vera Moisturizer, 358

S

Sadness and malaise
  Rose and Raspberry Jam, 288
Seasonal affective disorder
  (SAD), 288–289
  Uplifting Citrus Body Balm, 289–290
Shaving irritation
  Citrus, Sage, and Lavender
    Aftershave, 343–344
Sinus infection
  Rosemary–Tea Tree Sinus
    Treatment, 224–225
  Sinus Saver Formula, 225
Skin conditions. *See also* Acne;
    Dermatitis; Dry skin; Itchy, achy
    skin; Oily skin; Psoriasis; Residue
    and clogged pores; Skin irritation
  All-Purpose Calendula Salve, 359
  Aloe, Comfrey, and Lavender
    Soap, 359–360
  Boo-Boo Balm, 360–361
  Calendula Sunshine Bath Soak, 361–362
  Facial Steam, 362–363
  Rose Splash, 363–364
Skin irritation
  Comfrey and Calendula
    Skin Soother, 364
  Day-to-Night Liniment, 365

General Index

Acknowledgments

All through my years of herbal adventures, my sister, Maryanne Schwartz, has been by my side, usually dragging me into some new craft or skill. We have been such a team that many people who have taken classes from us or know us from various herbal functions just call us "the sisters" or, if they know us well, "the twisted sisters" from our old Renaissance festival days. Without her, I wouldn't have taken a fraction of the risks along the way. I wish that everyone could have such a great accomplice.

I'd also like to thank my editor, John Makowski, for his patience and helpfulness during the composition of this book.

About the Author

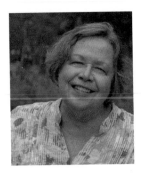 **Tina Sams** left the corporate world 30 years ago for her one true calling—plants. Twenty years ago, she dreamed up *The Essential Herbal* magazine. It has been a great joy to correspond with readers who become confident in their own use of herbs in medicine, food, gardening, and crafting. Various Essential Herbal social media outlets have worked as a hub to connect herbal enthusiasts who form deep friendships—one of her proudest accomplishments.

She and her sister travel around speaking about and teaching all sorts of herb skills, believing that sharing mistakes and foibles is as valuable as doing things correctly. "We make the mistakes so you don't have to" is their unofficial tagline.

Foraging wild plant foods, aromatic plant distillation, and natural dyeing are her favorite hobbies.